This

UMI
BOOKS ON DEMAND™

UMI
A Bell & Howell Company
300 North Zeeb Road • PO Box 1346
Ann Arbor, Michigan 48106-1346
800-521-0600 • 313-761-4700

MORALS AND MEDICINE

MORALS
AND MEDICINE

THE MORAL PROBLEMS OF:

The Patient's Right to Know the Truth
Contraception
Artificial Insemination
Sterilization
Euthanasia

By JOSEPH FLETCHER

WITH A FOREWORD BY KARL MENNINGER, M.D.

PRINCETON UNIVERSITY PRESS
PRINCETON, NEW JERSEY

To My Mother

CONTENTS

FOREWORD

UPPOSE the worst man in the world applied to the best surgeon in the world for relief from a condition that would prove fatal unless relieved by surgery. Should the surgeon operate? Suppose a man, while committing a murder, breaks a leg, but escapes immediate capture and applies to a doctor for relief? Should the doctor treat him? (Dr. Mudd, member of a distinguished American family, was given a long prison term for having done just this.) If an isolated doctor has ten patients, with enough serum to save five lives, which five shall he save? Or shall he run the risk of saving none by dividing it equally among them all?

These are not the questions in medical ethics with which Dr. Fletcher deals in this book, but they hint at the recurring problem of loyalty which arises over and over in the life of every practicing physician. Every doctor has loyalty, we may assume, to certain medical ideals, to certain social ideals, loyalty to the law of the land, loyalty to religious convictions, loyalty to his family. Conflicts in loyalty adherence are inevitable.

It is thus that a certain hierarchy of loyalties, a kind of graded value system, has to be set up by each individual. I have been consulted by Catholic priests and Protestant clergymen, by fellow psychiatrists and surgeons, by lawyers and judges who have said in an agony of spirit, "I don't know what I should do. I don't know what is the most nearly right thing to do." For no man can be entirely consistent, even to his own system, or entirely loyal to all of his loyalties. I recall hearing the greatest living man, Albert Schweitzer, in discussing his principle of reverence for life, say, with a sweet, sad smile, "But you see, I am not consistent; I decline meat, yet I am very fond of eggs."

Dr. Fletcher has examined the ethical problems and the

value systems of physicians, in the light of our Judaeo-Christian culture. In addition to certain broad general considerations, five practical problems in the ethics of medical practice are analyzed: These are the truthful communication of findings to the patient, regulation of conception, artificial insemination, sterilization, and euthanasia. Dr. Fletcher has limited himself to these questions of the physician's responsibility in matters of life and death in the course of medical practice, carefully eliminating such secondary problems as the tolerance of medical incompetence, the sadistic destruction of hope and the various complications involved in setting a monetary value on the techniques of saving life. He has tried—and, I think, successfully—to formulate a philosophy for the practical guidance of the physician.

Personality, he concludes, is not created by divine fiat but by a divinely ordained process of development. God is indeed the Maker of man, but only indirectly. The concept of the soul in the ordinary sense only contributes to the tendency of natural positivism and determinism to undermine ethics and ethical responsibility. "Biology cannot provide the content of theology." Living by spiritual standards is more valuable than life maintained at the cost of demoralization and depersonalization.

That the author is deeply religious and earnestly ethical no one can doubt. Some of his conclusions will be contrary to prevalent Roman Catholic convictions. Notwithstanding this, the author declares that "were medical workers and non-Catholics to expend the care and concern we have seen in the studies of the Roman theologians, how much might be gained for man's moral stature and for the claims of mercy and well-being! With the one stellar exception of Catholic moralists, there is a strange blindspot about the ethics of health and medicine in almost all ethical literature. Volume after volume in general ethics and in religious treatises on morality will cover almost every conceivable phase of personal and social ethics *except medicine and health*. It is high time that we brought our ethical and spiritual experience, and its new dimensions of understanding, to bear upon the care of the sick in the same deliberate and creative way that psychology has been explored and applied for the sake of those who are ill and in need of counsel and treatment."

The earnestness, the scholarliness, the conscientiousness and the thoroughness of the author cannot but appeal to scientists, philosophers and men of good will, even when their convictions and personal value system of hierarchies would lead them to differ in their conclusions. A great contribution has been made here to philosophy, to religion, to morality and to medicine.

KARL A. MENNINGER, M.D.

PREFACE TO
THE PRINCETON PAPERBACK EDITION

When this book first appeared in 1954, a quarter of a century ago, I complained that ethics had a "blind spot" because it dealt vigorously with personal morality and social problems but ignored questions of right and wrong in biology, medicine, and health care. That charge has no basis in fact anymore. A quick scan of the literature of ethics in the past decade shows not only the emergence of "bioethics" or "biomedical ethics" to a sophisticated degree but that it occupies an almost faddish place in the sun.

This course of development has managed to achieve a qualitative as well as a quantitative change. For the most part, especially in professional circles, medical ethics had always focussed on medical manners and deportment and on the physician's guild obligations. As a mode of treatment this tended to be either trivial or moralistic and sententious (with its warnings about not smelling of wine or tobacco, not sitting on the patient's bed, always obeying the Association's rules, and the like), or else it was couched in the language of pretty highflown idealism. That classical professional ethic has become in the past twenty-five years a mature ethical analysis of both medicine and its biological foundations. The questions it examines come home directly or indirectly to everybody, which makes it now an ethics *for* society and the patient population, rather than *of* the medical profession.

Perhaps *Morals and Medicine* got this process moving. Some have said so. It remained the only work of its kind for another fifteen years or more. To be sure, there was within the Catholic church a thorough and carefully systematic way of handling the issues posed by medical practice, even though its mode of weighing them was authoritarian and based on its own peculiar premises. (In point of fact, that system has managed to mature and relax in some significant respects.)

Indeed, when people have taken me to task occasionally for "always quarreling with the Catholics" (always is, of course, too strong), I have had to be at pains to point out that since theirs was the only adequate work in the field at that time, anything the rest of us did would have to take account of their moral theologians and acknowledge the weight of their formulations, even when we found their syllogisms did not stand up. Any serious discussion, aiming at more light and less heat, owes a special debt to those whose clearcut conclusions sharpen up the issues, even if the end result is disagreement.

The half-dozen problems the book explores are still being debated, and it may well be that no complete consensus can ever be reached about them. Nevertheless, patients' rights, truth-telling in medical diagnosis, and birth control (at least contraceptively, if not by sterilization and abortion) have found general acceptance. Even in the matter of voluntary euthanasia some real measure of a "changed mind" is evident. Eight states in the U.S. as of this date have already passed bills giving legal backing to Living Wills (directives to stop treatment in terminal illnesses), and more are sure to come.

When the book was first published I thought it would take a lot longer to reach this point than it has. Artificial insemination, like euthanasia, has had legal enactment in several states and is practiced everywhere anyway. *All* states have accepted voluntary sterilization. Law or no law, however, these things remain problematic and disputed in the hearts and minds of many people.

As far, at least, as my own thinking is concerned there is one element in this book which I have found no reason to change at all. I mean its basis or rootage in persons, in human beings, as the first-order value or highest good by which to make ethical appraisals. (That is, ideological or absolutized taboos ought not to be one's standard.) I am still convinced that what helps people individually or collectively is right, what hurts is wrong. Human benefit, I would want to contend, is the talisman of ethical propriety and justifies whatever we do, not only in biomedical ethics but in all questions of right and wrong, good and evil, desirable and undesirable—straight across the board of conscience and its problems. Such a humanistic ethics is appropriate as much to religious moralities as to a secular outlook.

In this last quarter of a century we have seen ethics follow an interesting pattern of development through four science-oriented phases. When *Morals and Medicine* appeared it was still the case that in normative ethics (problem-solving) we were largely tied to the social sciences; we felt, correctly enough, that ethics had a lot to learn from economics, political science, and sociology. Next we turned to the behavioral sciences: we wanted more light on ethical concepts such as motive, freedom, will, intention, determinism, and value selection. (Some of what we learned was sobering; it took the starch out of a lot of moralism and the conventional wisdom.)

In the third phase, triggered by the nuclear breakthrough, we looked at the physical sciences, but only to find tl.at our training in the humanities had not fitted us to grasp very fully a lot of physics and chemistry. In spite of this block we were alerted, and needfully so, to *technology's* credits and debits when its impacts are put in the scales of value judgment and choice; this, by the way, includes the "soft" technologies of medicine. Finally, in the late Sixties and Seventies ethics started to explore the biological front—the life sciences. This, of course, was what *Morals and Medicine* had pointed towards in 1954. Dealing not only with long-standing but also with newly emerging (but debatable) controls and manipulations of birth, health, and death is now the growing edge of normative ethics as a whole.

We can leave it there, I think, without either shirking known questions or inviting the hazards of futurizing. Sufficient unto the day are the good and evil thereof.

Belmont, Massachusetts
December 1978

JOSEPH FLETCHER

PREFACE (1954)

THIS book is about certain problems of conscience, certain ethical issues, which arise in the course of medical care. I have not dealt with medical ethics in the usual sense of those words. More commonly the phrase means merely a body of rules to govern the social behavior and graces of physicians. Neither have I entered into the technical merits of medical theories and practices, nor taken up various philosophies of health, life, and death as they are to be found in different parts of the world. Furthermore, there are almost innumerable cases of conscience in the whole range of medical care, but I have tried to explore only a few of the kind we might call the problems of *crisis* in life and death.

Inevitably, at least in our Western society, a discussion of right and wrong, of good and evil, in medical care will take us into questions relating to the Christian faith. Yet even here I have not attempted to construct or suggest a theology of medicine, as distinct from its ethics. Such a theology is needed according to Daniel Jenkins, who has gone so far as to assert, "To say that a theology of medicine is needed may sound pretentious, but something like it is necessary if Christian doctors are to understand their duty clearly."[1] He must have meant a *Protestant* theology, of course, for there is already a well-turned one, both explicit and implicit, in Catholic moral theology under the headings of the Fifth, Sixth, and Ninth Commandments. To my knowledge, nothing of this kind has been undertaken by non-Catholics as yet, and certainly this book is at the most only a modest contribution to the *ethics* of medicine, not to its theology. I hope, of course, that the ethical judgments I have reached are within the range and provision of Christian theology, but that would be all that could be claimed for them.

[1] *The Doctor's Profession*, London, 1949, p. 16.

The bias of my ethical standpoint, apart from its frame of reference in Christian faith, is probably best pin-pointed as personalist. It is not naturalist, humanist, hedonist, utilitarian, or positivist. As will be seen, by personalism I mean the correlation of personality and value; the doctrine, that is, that personality is a unique quality in every human being, and that it is both the highest good and the chief medium of our knowledge of the good. But it is better to let the meaning of these abstract terms become apparent as they are worked out in their application to the morals of medicine in the following pages.

At no time have I ever meant to take the position, or to give any comfort to those who would like to assume, that the clergy or other moralists can or should settle problems of medical conscience *for* the doctors. If doctors undertake to care for the health of our people, they must undertake to do it conscientiously. This is to say that they have to put their consciences to work, as they do their skills. Nothing could be more subversive of medical integrity, nor more irresponsible ethically, than the excuse once offered by an official of the American Academy of General Practice for hoping that a recent episode of medical euthanasia could be kept quiet and unmentioned at a convention. He said, "There are extremists on both sides. They will bring to the floor emotions more than anything else. The subject is emotional at present. *It is a moral question, not a scientific one. It is a matter for the church, not for doctors. We have other fish to fry.* I shall do everything possible to keep it out of the congress of delegates."[2] But nobody's opinions are any better than his facts. Physicians have an *expertise* and competence without which all non-medical discussion of the rights and wrongs of medicine will be in danger of becoming only wool-gather-

[2] *The New York Times*, Feb. 21, 1950. Italics added. Gerald Heard writes as if the solution of these problems were solely the doctors' responsibility: *Morals since 1900*, New York, 1950, p. 216.

ing. Of course there is emotion at work! This is true, perforce, in matters of life and health and death. It could not, humanly speaking, be otherwise. But to attempt, perhaps out of motives that do the medical profession very little credit, to draw watertight compartments between moral and scientific questions, especially when the science is related to so vital an art for people as is medicine, is to falsify reality beyond all possible tolerance. Medicine and human beings have suffered enough in the past because there were religionists who liked to say, and doctors willing to let them say, that morals in medicine are "a matter for the church, not for doctors." This book is a serious effort to expose the cynicism revealed in all protests that practitioners of the healing art have other fish to fry when it comes to conscience around the sick bed. Such cynicism accounts, perhaps, for the significant fact that the catalogues of medical libraries in this land turn up a great many titles on medical ethics written in the nineteenth century, but relatively few for the twentieth.

Many times throughout these pages I was tempted to illustrate the problems under examination by recounting experiences of my own. These experiences have been gained throughout a quarter of a century in the ministry, fifteen of them concentrated in the teaching and clinical supervision of theological students exploring human needs in parishes, hospitals, social agencies, and homes. The temptation to use my own case histories, even though this was often justifiable, I have steadfastly resisted.

The invitation to deliver the Lowell Lectures at Harvard University, for which the substance of this book was prepared in 1949, caused me some hesitation. First, I was reluctant to mount a foundation platform including such illustrious figures as Louis Agassiz, Bertrand Russell, Alfred North Whitehead, Amy Lowell, and others of a brilliance and ability so far beyond my own. Again, I was daunted more than a little because the lecture was described by its founder as not a popular one but of a "more erudite and particular" sort. I was afraid my purposes and hopes lay in just the other direction. But perhaps most of all, although I wanted keenly to explore the problems of morals and medicine, I felt some reluctance to attempt it because, apart from the work of Catholic scholars, the field had neither been explored in a systematic way nor broken down into manageable parts by earlier inquiries. The provision made in John Lowell's will of 1832 (written on the banks of the Nile as he sat "gazing in awe" at the old world ruins of Thebes) was that the lecturers should believe in "the divine revelation of the Old and New Testaments."[3] Although this requirement is presumably no longer enforced, it gave me at least one ground upon which I felt I could claim fitness for the venture.

It can only be said that this book shows the way to a field of ethical inquiry clamoring for attention, but too long neglected. In fact, I am the first to confess that it also illustrates, by its failures and defects, the difficulties of the task, and the continuing need of devoted and skillful investigation. There are some problems, such as the ethics of psychosurgery, not touched on at all. It is a matter for wonder that the philosophers have had so little to say about the physician and his medical arts. Indeed, they have said practically nothing as compared to the pronouncements of lawyers, scientists, businessmen, and citizens in general. I have never been content to note the fact as a fact, however, and leave it there. Mark Twain used to complain that while everybody talked about the weather, nobody ever seemed to do anything about it. I have done *something* about this matter, however incompletely and tentatively.

To my many friends in both medicine and morals, none of whom would be pleased in any way by personal mention,

---

[3] *Dict. of Amer. Biog.*, and H. K. Smith, *History of the Lowell Lectures*, Boston, 1898.

PREFACE (1954)

I am indebted for much sympathy, correction, and frank commentary on what I have written. Numbered among them are Catholics, Protestants, and non-religious idealists. For my mistakes I myself take the blame, which is only proper and even essential to the conception of ethical responsibility which runs as a central theme throughout these pages. It is an actual fact that this book would never have seen the light of day had it not been for my wife's persistence and belief that it has interest for others besides the author.

J.F.F.

Cambridge, Massachusetts
June 6, 1954

ACKNOWLEDGMENTS

GRATEFUL acknowledgment for permission to quote material from other publications is extended to the following: McIntosh and Otis, Inc., *American Freedom and Catholic Power*, by Paul Blanshard; Harper & Brothers, *Physician, Pastor, and Patient*, by G. W. Jacoby, and *Ends and Means*, by Aldous Huxley; MD Publications, Inc., for material by A. L. Woolbarst, in the *Medical Record*; Benziger Brothers, Inc., publishers and copyright owners, *Cases of Conscience*; Morehouse-Gorham Co. and the Society for the Promotion of Christian Knowledge, *The Christian Faith*, by C. B. Moss; Macmillan & Company, Ltd., *The Idea of Christian Atonement*, by Hastings Rashdall; *The New England Journal of Medicine*, "The Theology of Medicine," by Robert B. Osgood; International Publishers, *Handbook of Marxism*, edited by E. Burns; The Macmillan Company, *Honesty*, by Richard C. Cabot; the Catholic Hospital Association, *Ethical and Religious Directives; The Linacre Quarterly*, for material by Hilary R. Werts.

MORALS AND MEDICINE

CHAPTER ONE

HUMAN RIGHTS IN LIFE, HEALTH,
AND DEATH

Ethics and Medical Care

MEDICINE and religion have always been closely associated, until comparatively recent times. Long after the disappearance of the primitive medicine man or priestly witch doctor the alliance still continued as a self-conscious and openly embraced affair. It was a long journey from the savage belief that the diseases afflicting men had a divine origin and served as punishment, hex, or magic (the art of healing therefore being a priestly task) to the blunt opinion of Martin Luther that "no malady comes from God."[1] Their marriage in the past ceased to be completely harmonious once medical studies and practice began to assert a certain measure of scientific independence of both religion and priestcraft. But for a long while they were like "an ancient Romulus and Remus, suckled at the lugs of a common wolf mother, the superstitious fears of the people."[2] Even in modern America, only one generation before our own, it was not impossible to read on a rabbi's card, left on the table of a hospital waiting room, "Weddings and circumcisions respectfully solicited." Indeed, so ancient is our up-to-dateness that medical specialization first began among the priests, for in the fifth century B.C. each Egyptian physician treated a single disorder under a divine (polytheist) charter, and the early Romans (before the Greeks won their prestige) had a deity for each disease. "Even the itch was not without its goddess," they used to say.

[1] *Table Talk*, ed. William Hazlitt, Philadelphia, 1868, pp. 250-257.
[2] G. W. Jacoby, *Physician, Pastor and Patient*, New York, 1936, p. 75.

If we press the analogy of marriage as between medicine and religion, then we must recognize their divorce. Perhaps a better analogy is separation, a separation, however, which has not led to complete alienation. Perhaps they never come together anymore in the common bed of faith, but at least they face each other frequently in the drawing room of morals. Ethical values, morals and conscience, right and duty, the pursuit of life's store, simple existence itself—these matters are still common to both medicine and religion. In many more ways than most people suspect, not excluding physicians and clergymen themselves, medicine and religion have conscience and its claims at stake and in their keeping. We need not argue any longer, as Aristotle once did, whether moral law or medicine is nobler; whether it is a higher goal to make men virtuous or to make them sound of health. (Plato stated the position typically, putting morality before health.[3]) In our times we have come to understand that the two go together, each a buttress for the other. This much at least is made clear in the fundamentals of modern psychosomatic medicine, whatever may be its future course of development. A few men felt the marriage was still valid even on the threshold of modern times. One Giles Fermen, a physician of Ipswich in the Massachusetts Colony, for example, wrote about 1650: "I am strongly sett upon to study divinitie, my studies else must be lost: for physick is but a meene helpe." Later he went back to England and took holy orders.[4]

The very first medical treatise published in America, and the only one to appear in the seventeenth century, was written by a clergyman of Boston in 1677. The Reverend Thomas

---

[3] The *Laws*, Book One, the Athenian stranger. This issue persisted for a long time. L. Thorndike (*Science and Thought in the Fifteenth Century*, New York, 1929, p. 24) cites a tract by "Collucio Salutati" written in Florence in 1399 which repeats the classical argument that moral philosophy deals with the rational soul while medicine deals only with the body.

[4] S. A. Green, *History of Medicine in Massachusetts*, Boston, 1881, p. 31.

Thatcher, first minister of the Old South Church, wrote a broadside describing smallpox and urging its quarantine as a moral obligation upon both individuals and the community. In the early decades of the next century his precedent was followed by Cotton and Increase Mather, and by fellow parsons who gave moral support to Dr. Zabdiel Boyleston, then making "scandalous" inoculation experiments in which his own son was a guinea pig. Their moral defense of inoculation roused a storm of popular excitement and protest, ending in the destruction by arson of the first hospital for inoculation at Cat Island, Marblehead, in 1773.[5] Such is the technical specialism of our own times, two and a half centuries later, that no non-medical writer would (or should) attempt to follow Mr. Thatcher into the field of medicine, even though we still claim the right to invade the ethics of medical care. Whether fireworks will result when we do, remains to be seen.

It would be well to be quite clear about the scope of this inquiry. We are dealing with the *ethics of medical care*. This means we are *not* dealing with medical ethics, a term which is usually used for the rules governing the social conduct and graces of the medical profession. The American Medical Association, in its *Principles of Medical Ethics*, has formulated the essential rules of the fraternity. They are not elaborate. Medical ethics is the business of the medical profession, although certainly it has to fall somewhat within the limits of social obligation. The literature on professional medical conduct is relatively sparse. Dr. Richard C. Cabot declared in 1926 that he knew "of no medical school in which professional ethics is now systematically taught."[6] That situation remains in force in pretty much the same degree today, except in the Catholic medical schools. The most

[5] *Ibid.*, p. 58.
[6] *Adventures on the Borderlands of Ethics*, New York, 1926, ch. on "Ethics and the Medical Profession," pp. 23-55.

5

consistent treatment of the subject, based upon experience of a high order, is to be found in the George Washington Gay Lectures delivered from time to time at the Harvard Medical School. To be quite frank, a typical discussion of medical ethics is not a very serious or challenging enterprise in moral judgment. The extant literature on it consists for the most part in homilies on the bedside manner and such calculated questions of propriety and prudence as shined shoes, pressed trousers, tobacco odors, whether to drink Madeira, and the avoidance of split infinitives! It is composed, in a phrase, of manuals or exhortations on competitive success.[7]

Dr. George Jacoby gives medical ethics a somewhat loftier definition. He has expressed the view that it deals with "the question of the general attitude of the physician toward the patient: to what extent his duty obligates him to intervene in the patient's interest, and what demands the physician has a right and duty to make upon the patient's relatives in regard to obedience and subordination for the purposes of treatment."[8] Dr. Jacoby's use of such essentially ethical terms as "right" and "duty" brings us much closer to what we mean by "the ethics of medical care," as distinguished from medical (professional) ethics. But first it is worth our while to take full note of Dr. Jacoby's words: nowhere among them is there anything about what demands the *patient* has "a right and duty to make" upon his physicians. It is from this other perspective, from the patient's point of view, that we shall try in this book to examine the morals, principles, and values at stake in medical care.

[7] "The Role of Ethical Conduct in the Successful Medical Career," F. H. Washburn, M.D., *New England Journal of Med.*, 204.27, pp. 1141-1151.

[8] *Op.cit.*, p. 25. He says further, "the physician is not in a position to command or control, but can merely advise. He can advise authoritatively but beyond that he has no powers. Only in a few instances is his authority unlimited. This is the case when a patient lies on the operating table under anesthesia, or when a person suffering from mental disorder has been legally committed to an institution licensed for the care of such patients."

We are not to suppose that doctors are tyrants or megalomaniacs. These maladies operate as occupational hazards in other professions as often as in medicine. Professional medical ethics in this country has come a long way from the attitude expressed in the American Medical Association's code of 1847, in which it was urged that the physician should "study . . . to unite condescension with authority" because "reasonable indulgence should be granted to the mental imbecilities and caprices of the sick."[9] There is very little disposition (or possibility) of preserving what Dr. Cabot once called rather shortly the "old tradition of aristocratic, benevolent autocracy in medicine."[10] On the contrary, with the advances we have made in the psychology of therapeutic relationship there is today a general understanding that a person-centered approach to illness is superior to the problem-centered approach, and consequently the doctor's work is more deliberately predicated upon "the recognition of the worth of human personality" and its rights.[11] A hundred and fifty years ago the English physician Parry said that it is more important to know what manner of man has the disease than to know what disease he has.[12] After all, it might not be stretching logic too far to say that the spirit of the modern age would reverse the old anti-medical saw, "The operation was a success but the patient died." Recent developments in the dynamics of medical care would almost be content with, "The patient was a success, but the operation failed." Most dictionaries recognize that the word "patient" comes from *pati*, to suffer or endure; suffering is a personal experience, and therefore a primary factor in illness. It raises the physician's problem from a merely technical one to the level of moral and spiritual values. Sir William Osler said that

[9] Cited, Cabot, *Adventures* . . . , *op.cit.*, p. 39.

[10] *Honesty*, New York, 1938, p. 151.

[11] "Factors Influencing Ethical Concepts and Ideals among Medical Students," *Journal of the Amer. Med. Assoc.*, 113.1267-1270.

[12] Alfred Friedlander, M.D., *Journal of the Amer. Med. Assoc., ut supra.*

7

medical care is founded on the age-old desire of man to help his suffering brethren, a motive that makes the relationship of doctor to patient a moral one at bottom.

As Dr. Francis Peabody of the Boston City Hospital once told the Harvard medical students, "One of the essential qualities of the clinician is interest in humanity, for the secret of the care of the patient is in caring for the patient. . . . The treatment of a disease may be entirely impersonal; the care of a patient must be completely personal."[13] The moralist's interest in the ethics of medicine has to do with *the care of a patient*, not with the treatment of a disease. We are concerned with medical care rather than with medical treatment. Dr. Peabody's phrase captures the heart of the matter; the care of a patient "must be completely personal." And the person cared for is vastly more than a patient. "What is spoken of as a 'clinical picture' is not just a photograph of a man sick in bed; it is an impressionistic painting of the patient surrounded by his home, his relations, his friends, his joys, sorrows, hopes and fears."[14] What is this, but to say that a patient's moral and ethical rights and interests must weigh as heavily in the medical scales as his physical needs and condition?

Fatality versus Morality

What, to turn directly to our subject, *are* our human rights in health, life, and death to which the patient may lay claim? Health, life, and death are parts of a single continuous process of human existence. Life and death are the original and terminal points, and health lies in between them as our defense against "the thousand natural shocks that flesh is heir to." The *media vita* of the burial office in the Book of Common Prayer says that "in the midst of life

---

[13] *The Care of the Patient*, Cambridge, 1928, pp. 12 and 48.

[14] *Ibid.*, p. 15. As a pioneer insight, cf. R. C. Cabot, *Foregrounds and Backgrounds in Work for the Sick*, Boston, 1906.

we are in death," and this poetic way of putting it has full medical authority. Dr. Alfred Worcester has explained that "in point of fact we are always dying."[15] Health, life, and death are a continuum, a single web of being. In the nature of the case nothing is more decisive for us than life and death, being born and "giving up the ghost" again; nor is anything more precious than the health of mind and body which makes our passage between these two crises one of beauty and joy rather than of ugliness and crippled being. Too much of the time (as we shall see) these decisive events lie outside human consciousness and rational control, which is the *ethical* significance of Dr. Osler's remark, in an Ingersoll Lecture, that most people die as they were born, not knowing what is happening.

Medical care is provided for persons. As Paul Tillich says, " 'Person' is a moral concept, pointing to a being which we are asked to respect as the bearer of a dignity equal to our own, and which we are not permitted to use as a means for a purpose, because it is purpose in itself."[16] This is of course a restatement of Kant's second maxim, "Act so as to treat humanity, whether in thine own person or in the person of another, always as an end, never as a means only." If medicine is completely personal it takes account of our human rights. We have certain rights, each of us, in our health, life, and dying. Justice, the philosophers say, consists in giving to all their due, their rights, that to which they are entitled. And to what, exactly, are we entitled in being born, in seeking and keeping health, in dying and "shuffling off this mortal coil"? To answer Hamlet's question, none of us has it in his power, to begin with, to choose whether "to be or not to be."[17] Whether we are born at all or not lies entirely with others to decide, not with us. But whether we

---

[15] "The Care of the Dying," *Physician and Patient*, Cambridge, 1929, p. 201.
[16] *The Protestant Era*, ed. by James L. Adams, Chicago, 1948, p. 115.
[17] Act III, Scene 1. This soliloquy pin-pricks most of this book's problems.

shall *continue* to be, to live, and upon what terms of life and health we make our choice, these are matters in which we can exercise some freedom, some choice, as responsible creatures.

Choice and responsibility are the very heart of ethics, and the *sine qua non* of a man's moral status. While it is true that we have no responsibility for our own birth, and therefore no moral stake in it, we *do* have a moral stake in the conception and birth of others, of those whom we bring into this world as we ourselves were brought. Life, health, and death are therefore moral issues. We can "do something about them" and therefore we have to decide what to do. It is this fundamental truth about our human existence which sets us apart from the rest of the animal order: the fact that so much of our destiny is or may be a matter of deliberate decision, of rational conduct, rather than of merely instinctive behavior. The whole history of man's moral growth since what Breasted called "the dawn of conscience" and classical or old-fashioned theologians call (so curiously) "the Fall," has been our steady march upward in the scale of responsibility from predetermined to self-determined action, from customary to reflective or rational morality.[18] In moving beyond brute existence man (who is so much weaker physically than many of the vertebrates) has had only two biological advantages with which to emancipate himself from nature's irrational limits and habits. One, and the more important one, is the higher intelligence to help him choose between ends, as well as between means. The other is his upright carriage, which has freed his hands, and gained him his Greek genus-name *anthropos*, meaning "the one who walks with his face to the heavens."

[18] J. H. Breasted, *The Dawn of Conscience*, New York, 1934. It has been steadily upward in the secular or broad trend, although certainly not automatic or constant, either in the species or in the individual. Moral progress and *automatic* moral progress are not the same thing. The latter idea, a form of unrealistic complacency, is borne out neither by history nor clinical observation in our own times.

The dimensions of our moral responsibility expand, of necessity, with the advances made in medical science and medical technology. Almost every year brings with it some new gain in our struggle to establish control over health, life, and death. There are far fewer reasons for us, in this generation, to be fatalistic about these crucial episodes of our existence than there were for our forefathers. Fatalism, which reflects a lack of control, is the outlook of those who are helpless to prevent or to put an end to what *they might not choose had they the power of choice.* Just as helplessness is the bed-soil of fatalism, so control is the basis of freedom and responsibility, of moral action, of truly *human* behavior. A "human act" in ethical theory and moral theology is defined as one which is free and understanding, not limited invincibly by ignorance or constraint.[19] It is for this reason that science, in spite of its frequent tragic misuses, contributes to our moral range and the magnitude of our ethical life; technology not only changes culture, it adds to our moral stature. The "technology" of sex, as a part of medical care, illustrates the general rule. For example, prophylactic and contraceptive devices have eliminated the old restraints upon extramarital sexuality, the old triple terrors of conception, infection, and detection, which once held people in line. These risks are almost a thing of the past. Science tends to remove moral compulsions. This means, by a significant paradox, the moral responsibility is being *enhanced*; our moral stature is heightened. It may not seem so, at first sight, to those who learn that in the final stages of the Second World War the U.S. Army was giving out 50,000,000 individual prophylactics each month. Here is, admittedly, a measure of the promiscuity in our culture at the

---

[19] Cf. any classical treatment, e.g., Koch-Preuss, *Handbook of Moral Theology*, St. Louis, 1925, I, 253-255. John Dewey and J. H. Tufts, *Ethics*, New York, 1914, p. 201ff. Emil Brunner, *The Divine Imperative*, London, 1937, p. 82ff. Less systematic discussions, whether religious or not, all agree that freedom and knowledge are the postulates of moral acts.

level of military and official practice. There is no way to estimate it for the civil populace as a whole. The widely debated taxonomic studies of sexual behavior in the American male and female, made by Dr. Alfred C. Kinsey and his associates, are a big step in the direction of more exact knowledge of our sexual mores, and their findings to date certainly seem to confirm the view that heterosexual practices are not at all restricted to monogamous marriage. Nevertheless, when external sanctions such as fear of consequences are minimized by medicine, then our internal controls are thereby raised to a higher power of importance. And, of course, with every such increase of personal responsibility and free choice, the chances of moral failure are also increased. The fact of failure raises a problem of religious resources, of "grace" and moral strength, but that would be the subject of another book.

In any discussion of morals and medicine it becomes necessary to trace our moral freedom, our human action, in a number of decisions over life and death. It has to be done in such a way that these events are seen to be, or seen to be capable of becoming, true decisions and not mere biological fatalities. The point is sharpened by Dr. Karl Menninger, in his analysis of ways in which childhood resentments of the mother may become a cause of destructive aggressions later on. He says, "It is philosophically naïve to talk about personal causes, as distinguished from impersonal causes, because of course everything is related to, and in that sense *causes*, everything else; hence, we get nowhere by the antiquated sophistry of inquiring 'who is to blame.' Blame is a legal and religious concept, not a scientific one."[20] For our purposes here we may paraphrase by saying, "*Responsibility* is a legal and religious [i.e., ethical] concept, not an empirical one." Responsibility is not a matter of natural and objective fact; it is a moral and spiritual thing. It is a human and per-

[20] *Love Against Hate*, New York, 1942, p. 34.

sonal phenomenon, not to be found "out there" in the physical world.

With the medical technology of contraception, parenthood and birth have become questions of moral responsibility; we are able to control the incidence of fertility. No longer do we have to choose between reproduction *or* continence. Sex is no longer either a submission to biological consequences or a denial of sex itself, as in continence or in so-called rhythm methods of birth control as recommended by some Catholic moralists and church authorities. This form of freedom is, indeed, not true freedom at all; it is only an *alternation of necessities*, not a matter of human control. Over against the necessity of biological nature (conception) it sets either the necessity of complete abstention (continence) or the necessity of periodic abstention (rhythm). In either case, biology lays down the conditions, man does not. Rhythm, except for its sophisticated mathematics and lunar calculations, is as ancient and pre-scientific as the first primitive insight that connected intercourse with childbearing.[21] With the technology of sterilization, we are able to choose for or against fertility itself. Sterilization gives us decisive control over parenthood, makes it our responsibility whether to be parents at all. With the medical technology of artificial insemination, we are able even to transcend biological barriers, if we choose. Undesired, merely accidental sterility, in the case of the male partner, no longer determines for a couple whether the wife shall have "a child of her own," and he a child by free choice and vocation. Artificial insemination has made it, now, a matter of morality rather than of fatality. Indeed, it is possible even further to outwit sterility, or biologically barren love, by the transplantation of viable ova to a sterile female partner. As far as scientific know-how is concerned, a further reach of pos-

[21] H. A. Fallon, *Rhythm Calculator with Dial Calculator and Calendar*, R-C Pub. Co., 5341 Forest Street, Kansas City, Mo., 1945.

sibilities, however ridiculous its practice might seem for cultural reasons, lies in the fact that it is possible to combine the sperm and ova of husband and wife and transplant the fertilized egg to another woman as host for gestation, the child born having the inheritance of the father and mother and receiving from the proxy mother nothing but the necessary nourishment. No longer, in short, are we compelled to choose between a marriage found barren, and parenthood. And finally, by euthanasia, we are able to control our being or not being.

Up to this point it must seem that the real subject under examination is eugenics. However, if this is so, then our particular concern is the moral aspects of eugenics as a social policy. The popular use of eugenics obscures the scientific distinction between eugenics (healthy procreation of persons) and euthenics (the healthy procreation of populations), a social problem not immediately relevant to the ethics of medical care. It is the *former* field of interest to which we are turning our attention: eugenics only in the sense that we cannot tolerate cacogenics, however it might be defended as a natural or divine state of affairs. Our concern is with the rights and wrongs of controlling life itself; we have no direct interest here in the population rates of the secular trend, or in broad social policies of positive and negative regulation.[22] Eugenics has been said to be "the science of good breeding," and our problem throughout these pages will be to explore the morality of such matters as sex and

[22] For the scientific side, cf. F. Osborn, *Preface to Eugenics*, New York, 1940, and for the demographic approach, cf. W. Vogt, *Road to Survival*, New York, 1948. Catholic moralists usually oppose population control in their struggle against birth control. E.g., the Rev. Edgar Schmiedeler, director of the Family Life Bureau of the National Catholic Welfare Council, has no scruples against appealing to race and class prejudice and to war sentiment in a letter to *The Reader's Digest*, Oct. 1943. He says family limitation is a "menace to the future leadership of the white race" and quotes Theodore Roosevelt and Winston Churchill on "the danger of birth control to our working and fighting population." The same fears are often expressed by non-Catholics as well.

eugenics while remaining as loyal as possible to the demands of good breeding in Emily Post's sense of the words as well as in Sir Francis Galton's.

Furthermore, it might be well at the outset to make it clear that we will not deal with *every* moral question involved in health, life, and death. Our range is deliberately held to the level of personal morality, insofar as it may realistically be abstracted from social justice and public morality. For this reason we cannot attempt to discuss sanitation, for example, important as it is to individual health in the compact urban community. Capital punishment is certainly another moral issue of life and death, but it, too, is a question more of legal ethics and social morality. (At several points it is entirely relevant, as an analogy or parallel in ethical judgment.) But our interest will be focused upon those moral issues which are, or in our opinion ought to be, regarded by general consent as matters of private choice and responsibility.

Our Viewpoint Has a Counterpoint

Any serious exploration of morality and ethics is bound to pay its respects to the past record of opinion and practice. It is often said that the greatest cultural achievement of modern times, in our human effort to understand ourselves and the world in which we live, is our grasp of historical perspective.[23] We have a sense of development and we appreciate to how great an extent our present problems are illumined by knowledge of the past. Archbishop Temple held that "above all, we have acquired and inherited the historical point of view, which more than anything else is the real distinction of the modern mind."[24]

If we act on this principle, our attention will be turned at many junctures to religion, for the simple reason that

[23] J. H. Robinson, *The Mind in the Making*, New York, 1921.
[24] *Christianity and the State*, London, 1928, p. 27.

until comparatively recent times religion has been the chief framework and vehicle of morals and moral opinion. The observation that the past alliance of morals and religion has broken down for many modern Americans ought not to make us forget their past interaction. But they are not even today altogether unrelated, if only negatively too much of the time. Indeed, as we shall see, organized religion in the churches is sometimes one of the chief brakes upon our moral growth in medicine. It seeks at many points to reduce or confine the areas and limits of responsible choice which are, by a counterforce, being widened by medical skill. E. R. Goodenough, Professor of Religion at Yale University, told the American Association for Mental Deficiency, meeting in Boston in December 1948, that, "if churches oppose what seems the best scientific procedure they must be resisted and circumvented. Modern medicine must never forget that it got its start when it defied legal and ecclesiastical prejudice in England and the Continent by stealing corpses to dissect them when they could be got no other way."[25] Before we are finished we shall see that very much the same problem still exists, for organized religion exerts an influence upon the morality and freedom of medical care, and upon the honesty and responsibility of medical science.

Very probably the most important observation to make here is that Catholic literature on the morals of medical care is both extensive and painstaking in its technical detail, while Protestant and Jewish literature is practically non-existent. It is for this reason chiefly that much of our analysis of the morals and problems of conscience in medicine will find a kind of counterpoint in the Roman Catholic literature. It is to be hoped, of course, that theological or religious bias is eliminated from this use of Catholic discussions, but where it may seem to have crept in the honest reader will have to correct for it by his own sense of proportion and

[25] *The Churchman*, Jan. 15, 1949.

fair play. Perhaps there is even a genuine hope in Catholic circles that others may take these matters seriously, even though Protestantism is never likely to enact official directives. Dr. O'Malley says, "Decrees of the Catholic Church are cited . . . not because morality is an asset of the Catholic Church alone, but because it alone pronounces officially on these medical subjects after careful consideration by competent specialists."[26]

A study of the *Cumulative Book Index* and of the *International Index of Periodicals*, which bears out this difference in interest and moral analysis, provides the student of ethics with a surprising comparative measure of the interest of religionists in health, life, and death. The same thing is to be discovered in medical circles, where (as separate from the American Medical Association) there is a Federation of Catholic Physicians' Guilds, but no Protestant counterpart, and a *Linacre Quarterly*, a Catholic journal of the philosophy and ethics of medical practice, but nothing at all equivalent to it from a Protestant source.[27] Jewish doctors and scholars have an excellent medium in *The Hebrew Medical Journal*, although it does not attempt to provide a theological or ethical rationale in any degree as detailed as the Catholic publication.[28] It is true that Protestant *pastors* concerned with personal counselling and ministry to the sick have their *Journal of Pastoral Care*, but this is only by and for ministers of religion.[29] No fraternity of non-Catholic physicians exists, as such.

In a highly controversial book (and, it must be admitted, a somewhat tendentious one, for all its careful documenta-

[26] Austin O'Malley, *The Ethics of Medical Homicide and Mutilation*, New York, 1919, preface.

[27] 1402 So. Grand Blvd., St. Louis 4, Mo. Named for Thomas Linacre (1460-1524), a physician to the court of England, founder of the College of Medicine, and a clergyman.

[28] Semi-annual bilingual, 983 Park Ave., New York 28, N.Y.

[29] Pub. by the Council for Clinical Training, jointly with the Institute of Pastoral Care, at 1312 Eye St., N.W., Washington 5, D.C.

tion) Paul Blanshard has had this to say which bears upon the leading place now held by Catholics in the field of morals and medicine:

"Most Americans would be somewhat startled if they picked up a medical journal and read a table of contents like this:

> *Episcopal Principles of Therapeutic Abortion*, by Bishop Sylvanus Bump, D.D.
>
> *Baptist Technique for Removing Gall Bladders*, by James McCutcheon, S.T.D.
>
> *How a Methodist Nurse Should Behave in a Presbyterian Hospital*, by Deaconess Matilda Little, M.A.
>
> *Jewish Ideals and the Caesarian Operation*, by Rabbi Marcus Goldberg, Ph.D.

"Such a table of content, of course, is purely imaginary, but the actual titles of priestly articles on medicine in Catholic magazines are no less startling. Denominational excursions into the field of practical medicine are almost unknown among Protestants and Jews, but the homiletic and ecclesiastical journals of the American priesthood treat many medical problems as a branch of theology and discuss specific medical subjects with great authority. . . .

"The priests of the church are not only spiritual advisors to the Catholic physician and nurse, but they exercise definite authority over the doctor and nurse in respect to many aspects of professional life. This is particularly true in the special areas of birth, death, and sexual conduct."[30]

Aware that there are 692 Catholic general hospitals in the United States in which nurses and doctors are subject to the Roman medical code, and that 3,300,000 patients (most of them non-Catholics) are treated in these hospitals every year, Mr. Blanshard was, as a journalist, concerned only with the "medical dogmas which priests seek to impose upon

[30] *American Freedom and Catholic Power*, Boston, 1949, pp. 107-108.

American Catholics." He has singled out certain principles from their teachings, evidently because they are startling and rather sensational. They are: (1) "the equality of mother and fetus" (under which it follows that doctors must refuse to directly damage the fetus, whether viable or not, if a choice must be made between its integrity and the mother's life, regardless of circumstances); (2) "the doctrine of the sacred head" (from which it is deduced that a doctor may never perform a craniotomy at childbirth, even if it is necessary in order to save the mother and even if the child is a monster, because the soul of the fetus is equal to the mother's and the probable seat of the soul is in the head); (3) "the doctrine of ectopic pregnancy" (which allows no right to a surgical operation directly aimed at removing a misplaced fetus growing in the fallopian tubes instead of in the womb, even though the death of the mother and child alike will be practically certain under this rule); (4) "the doctrine of protection against heresy" (which forbids Catholic hospital personnel to call non-Catholic ministers for non-Catholic patients, even at their express request, since that would be to cooperate in the practice of a "false" religion).[31]

Now, as we shall see in some detail later on, Mr. Blanshard has chosen to shock his readers rather than to explain the tortuous and detailed arguments with which Catholic moralists handle these matters. The result is an inexact and incomplete account of the Catholic views. His exposition by no means takes sufficient account, even in the problems he

---

[31] This outline by Mr. Blanshard was first published in *The Nation*, Jan. 1, 1947, and then elaborated on pp. 111-131 of his book, *op.cit.* His second point, about the "sacred head," seems to be ungrounded. Roman Catholic moralists prohibit craniotomies because they are a direct killing of an unborn child, not because of any particular relation of the soul to the head. The same prohibition applies to evisceration of a fetus or the piercing of the heart. As for Blanshard's fourth point, a typical discussion is to be found in C. J. McFadden's *Medical Ethics for Nurses*, Philadelphia, 1946, p. 333: A nurse "may not encourage or assist" a patient to practice a non-Catholic faith, but she may ask a non-Catholic nurse to call a non-Catholic minister for non-Catholic patients.

selects, of the practical import of the Rule of Double Effect, nor of the distinction between direct and indirect damage or aggression, nor of the reluctant but relaxing casuistry that is developing among some moral theologians. A whole new dimension of possibilities is exposed to view in these timid but humble words of the English moralist, Father Davis: "The moralists who condemn the operation [of ectopic excision] must be very sure of their ground, for they are running counter to a large body of surgical opinion, in a matter that is confessedly obscure; they are asking the Catholic surgeon to run the risk of either relinquishing all such cases or retiring from his profession."[32] Furthermore, all these doctrines cited above are related primarily to the problem of abortion, but abortion is only one among the moral issues of health, life, and death with which this volume is concerned. There are many other questions of right and wrong in medical care upon which Catholic moralists have settled views, and in the determination of them they have played a pioneering role. To say less than this would be ungracious, at the very least. Whether or not those that follow the paths they have broken will agree with their conclusions is another matter. They are rather like the antiquarian, of whom Sir Walter Scott said that he was a very positive man, and like most positive men, he was sometimes right!

Our Problem Has a Past

Aesculapius, son of Apollo, like Imhotep in Egypt, is the legendary father of medicine. Apollo gave Hermes the caduceus (serpents twined on a staff) which is still the emblem of the medical art. Aesculapius, killed by a thunderbolt of Jove, had two children: Hygeia, who took the sponsorship of health, and Panacea, who took the sponsorship of medicine. In the Hippocratic Oath, which seems to date from about 400 B.C., it was laid down that physicians should be

[32] Henry Davis, S.J., *Moral and Pastoral Theology*, New York, 1943, II, 182.

"pious without going so far as superstition."[33] This gives us some idea of how far back into antiquity runs the tension between religion and medicine. Nicor, the father of Galen, is reputed to have warned his fellow physicians that "sects are implacable despots; to accept their thralldom is to take away all liberty from one's action and thought."[34] It is not clear, from his own words, whether Galen referred to medical or religious sects. His warning applies in either case. It is on just such grounds of ancient wisdom and of long and sometimes bitter experience that the American Medical Association insists that a physician should not base his practice on an exclusive dogma or sectarian system.[35] This principle becomes all the more pertinent and imperative when medical care finds itself involved in a systematic moral theology of the magnitude and reach of the Catholic scholars, covering, as it does, ethical judgments upon all details of physical life from the conception of life itself to post-mortem questions like cremation, the disposal of diseased organs and members, and even the kind of ground in which a body may be buried.

We can fully appreciate the ramifications and difficulties of such sweeping attempts to "theologize" medical care without following the hard opinion of Dean Inge, then of St. Paul's Cathedral in London, that religion is "a powerful antiseptic, which preserves mumified customs that have long outlasted their usefulness, and otiose dogmas that have long lost their authority"[36] Too often the Christian Church has tried to oppose or fetter many of medicine's chief powers. Merely as examples of this, we can recall that surgery and dissection—as in the Edict of Tours, A.D. 1163, which forbade the shedding of blood—were gravely hindered and even anathematized as subversive of the doctrine of the bodily

[33] *Principles of Medical Ethics*, A.M.A., 1940.
[34] *Ibid.*   [35] *Ibid.*
[36] Quoted. Jacoby, *op.cit.*, p. 90.

resurrection of Christ.[37] After the Reformation, theological restrictions were often even stricter. In 1638 the Rector of the University of Paris objected to granting a doctorate in medicine to a Protestant, insisting on the exclusion of all heretics from the candidates' classes.[38] In the end, of course, the church has always given in to the steady pressure of man's growing self-determination as his growing pains were fortified by the triumphs of medicine. As in the cases of surgery and dissection, so in other skills, one by one the church's battles against vaccination, vivisection, narcosis, anesthetics, inoculation, and many others, have ended in defeat. Ultimate capitulation in these matters has exemplified the old maxim of prudential morality, "if you cannot lick them, join them."

Curiously enough, there is very little about medicine and pharmacy in the Bible or in the Talmud. We can see there was a kind of ethos among the prophets which opposed them to the priests, and to their sacerdotalism with its rigid and fear-ridden tabu morality. The prophets were capable morally, if the priests were not, of understanding what Huxley meant by saying, "New truths begin as heresies and end as superstitions," a *bon mot* which applies to medicine as much as to religion.[39] To preserve a balance in the record, we should also be clear that Christian leadership has upon occasion in the past helped medical powers, not hindered them. Even in the Middle Ages there were clerical friends of medicine, such as the monk Bertharius of Monte Cassino, and Pope Honorius II, who established medical schools and assisted the art in every way. Gregory the Great and St. Bernard were champions of the faith who stood in the way of medical progress, but Clement III and Sylvester II gave

---

[37] *Ibid.*, p. 87. Cf. also B. J. Stern, *Society and Medical Progress*, London, 1941, pp. 177-179. Charles Singer, *Evolution of Anatomy*, London, 1925, p. 85f., disagrees with the view of most historians that the bull of Boniface VIII in 1300, *De sepulturis*, was used to block dissection.

[38] Stern, *op.cit.*, p. 83.   [39] *Ibid.*, p. 152.

it aid and comfort.[40] This was in the days before the Fourth Lateran Council, at which priests were forbidden by canon law to carry on the practice of medicine unless they had an "indult" from the Holy See permitting them to give "physick" or surgical services. One wonders, nevertheless, whether there are not a good many Christians even today who would still agree, deep down, with John of Arezzo, who warned Lorenzo de Medici that the practice of medicine is under the rule of Mars and Scorpion, signs and planets which are "invidious, malevolent, plotting and hating all others."[41]

Religions other than Christianity and Judaism have often shown a more direct intervention in medicine and exerted a more superstitious influence. In China, of the 72 Buddhas, 29 are gods of healing or of drugs; in Taoism, of 150 particular hells one is reserved for physicians (very much as Dante, in his *Inferno*, reserved one at the nethermost level for bankers.[42]) It is a notorious fact in Christian missions that Hinduism regards childbirth as unclean, so that missionaries have to work with great tact to overcome this attitude, in much the same spirit with which they have had to overcome the popular Western interpretation of Psalm 51, "Behold I was shapen in wickedness, and in sin hath my mother conceived me." *Charakha*, an Indian medical code of about A.D. 100, is in a striking degree more tabu-bound than its Western counterpart, the Hippocratic Oath.[43] The role of the witch doctor or the medicine-priest is great or small in direct proportion to a religion's primitive quality, culturally speak-

[40] Cf. A. D. White, *Hist. of the Warfare of Science with Theology*, New York, 1897, II, 35-36. White appears to begrudge any credit to medieval Christians. At the opposite extreme is J. J. Walsh's *The Catholic Church and Healing*, New York, 1928.

[41] L. Thorndike, *op.cit.*, p. 57. This suspicion could be held of some orthodox Christians, and not only of sectarian doctrines and heterodoxies like Christian Science.

[42] C. H. Wall, *The Curious Lore of Drugs and Medicine*, New York, 1927, pp. 357-358.

[43] Cf. F. C. Shattuck, "Medical Ethics," an address at Western Reserve Medical College, Apr. 25, 1908.

ing. Yet there has been and still is in Christendom enough culture lag between medicine and religion to pose a serious problem. We have quoted Luther's view that "no malady comes from God," a saying in which he was following St. Augustine's opinion. It was not uttered in a modern or scientific spirit of medical materialism or as a theory of natural (physical) causation. The Bishop of Hippo had held that all diseases of Christians are due to demons who especially attack freshly baptized children and adults, "yea, even the guiltless, newborn infants."[44] The English *Book of Common Prayer* seemed, shortly after Luther's time, more willing to attribute physical evil to God's doing than to preserve St. Augustine's demonology; it said (and still does, in the Exhortation) that we ought not "to kindle God's wrath" or "provoke him to plague us with divers diseases and sundry kinds of death." The American church, we may be grateful to note, delicately left out that passage when it set up its own version. As we shall see, this kind of superstitious etiology and the theocratic morality attached to it is still widespread among us, even in the middle of the twentieth century.

The Book of Ecclesiasticus, not a part of the Protestant canonical Holy Scriptures, but nevertheless sometimes read in churches, has this to say: "Honor a physician according to thy need of him: for verily the Lord hath created him. . . . My son, in thy sickness be not negligent; but pray unto the Lord, and he shall heal thee. . . . Then give place to the physician, for verily the Lord hath created him; and let him not go from thee, for thou hast need of him. *There is a time when in their very hands is the issue for good.*"[45] This quotation from the wisdom of Jesus the son of Sirach, in the King James or Authorized Translation, supplies an appropriate text for the thesis of this book. Perhaps the writer meant

[44] Quoted A. D. White, *op.cit.*, ii, 27; *De Divinatione Daemonum*, iii (xl, Migne, 585).
[45] 38.1-15. Italics added.

safety of health, rather than moral rectitude, when he spoke of "the issue for good," but whichever way it was meant it is true that "good" in both senses often lies in the hands of the physician, to be done or denied. This is certainly the case when the patient's right to know the truth about his condition is in question, or when it comes to the patient's right to control parenthood by contraception, or to cease reproducing by means of sterilization, or to overcome childlessness by artificial insemination, or to die by euthanasia. "There is a time when in their hands is the issue for good."

Our Problem Has a Future

In the chapters to follow we shall attempt, as reasonably as may be, to plead the ethical case for our human rights (certain conditions being satisfied) to use contraceptives, to seek insemination anonymously from a donor, to be sterilized, and to receive a merciful death from a medically competent euthanasiast. We believe we can show, at the very least, that any *absolute* prohibition of these boons of medicine is morally unjustified, subversive of human dignity, and most serious of all, spiritually oppressive. These matters are neither academic in character nor infrequent in their practical occurrence as questions of conscience in medical care and human experience. The fact that when they do occur they are often hushed up, by a timid conspiracy of patient and doctor overawed by customary morality, neither reduces their frequency nor diminishes their moral importance. The morbidity rate of tragedies transmissible by inheritance, the alarming incidence of sterility among adults wanting children of their own, and the pathetic prevalence of terminal diseases such as cancer, are probably far more common than most of us realize. In the case of cancer, for example, we must begin to reckon soon, and honestly, with the consequences of medicine's success in prolonging our life-expectation. Most people are agreed that medicine's proper purpose

25

is to prolong life. That being so, what will happen now that medicine has so well served its goal that one man out of eight or ten, and one woman in six, will have to go under the knife, the radium pack, or the X-ray tube because a dangerous, often irresistible growth takes possession of the body? The mortality rate for cancer has nearly doubled in the past thirty years. During 1950 about 210,700 people died of it in the United States alone. This increase is directly due to the fact that medicine is prolonging life to the point where these tumors can occur frequently and develop rapidly. Paradoxically, this is a fruit of medical success! Moralists who spend little or no time in the terminal wards of a modern city hospital cannot contribute much in the way of realistic opinion or relevance on the subject of euthanasia. They need to examine the facts, or to re-examine them, not only statistically but clinically.

The ethics of medical care have to change, to grow, and to engage constantly in self-correction. This is true because medicine is a human art for human beings, and we human beings increase in wisdom and stature, even as the Son of Man did.[46] When we are tempted to despair over the inertia of the common run in the face of new moral challenges, we can always find reassurance by remembering that the culture progression from Neanderthal man persisted, to the desert man on the edge of the Hittite world, then to the medieval villein, then to the citizen of a modern democracy. This is the sequence, in part, a story of moral progress, progress in two fundamental respects. It is seen, first, in *the individuation of men from the tribal group*, the emergence of true personal integrity or being; and, second, in *the control men have gained over their circumstances*, which is the basis of their freedom. Personal integrity and freedom are the heart and muscles of morality. They come slowly, sometimes painfully. Never is the ideal of what is good and what is

[46] Luke 2:52.

26

right once for all delivered to the saints, or entirely plain to us in its full requirement. The history of the ethics of medical care is dramatic proof of these things—of morality as a process rather than a given quantity, as a contingency of freedom, as an acknowledgment of self-determination and of personal worth.

Problems of conscience in medicine are in a sense created by progress in four distinguishable phases of medical growth. We can state them very briefly in this way: (1) *changes in technology*, which precipitate conflicts of value and sentiment such as those between the personal ministrations of the general practitioner on the one hand, and the efficient but relatively impersonal specialization (and therefore collectivization) of practice in and out of hospitals, on the other hand; (2) *professional experience,* raising such questions of prudence as whether to use the new lobotomies for some of the psychoses, since it is alleged that the patient sometimes undergoes personality regressions or changes; (3) *scientific advances*, which introduce doubts as to whether medical researchers who are also physicians, under the Hippocratic Oath to fight illness and pain, should, for example, turn over their knowledge of botulisms to militarists for bacteriological warfare; and (4) *cultural changes*, which raise for doctors such questions as whether their first loyalty, which has always been to the patient, is in any way compromised or diluted by engaging in contract or group practice for a union or a firm or a government, in order to minister to a defined but not an individualized clientele.[47] The moral problems of medicine are almost always a mixture of several of these developments. Further, we ought to take notice that these ethical questions seem to take their shape under the pressures of three other factors at work: (a) *the spread of psychology*

[47] This fourth source is well discussed in Joseph Laufer, "Ethical and Legal Restrictions on Contract and Corporate Practice of Medicine," *Law and Contemporary Problems*, Oct. 1939, 4.4.

and its application to medical practice, as in the question whether physicians should withhold the truth from their patients when psychotherapy shows that "ignorance is bliss," and that self-knowledge is sometimes destructive; (b) *the economics of medical care*, as in the values at stake in any conversion to group practice, voluntary industrial and group insurance, and in programs of socialized medicine and panel practice; and (c) *interference with medical practice* by old religious beliefs and customary morality. All of these things have a bearing, but somehow the last-named factor seems to crystallize them all, for purposes of ethical analysis.

Although enough has been said about old religious beliefs for our present purposes, we shall have to cope with them in detail later on because of their persistence in specific moral issues. However, a few more things might be said here about customary morality. First of all, we should clearly distinguish it from reflective or rational morality, and from theocratic or revealed morality. The primitive personality, whether of the past or of the present, bases his moral opinions on custom, on group habit, accepting them without much reflection. His moral impulse is to "keep up with the Joneses" and, for his ethical subsistence he lives on the cake of custom. Customary morality is also subject to the rule of change, but it changes slowly with changes in social convention, *without personal choice or decision*. The margin of freedom and self-determination is relatively small. It condemns the traditional evils, remains blind to the new and emergent wrongs. It works well in a stable environment; but when conditions are changing its weaknesses show up, however reluctant or even hysterical its addicts may be in coming to terms with the new reality situation. As Dean Hodges of the Episcopal Theological School said to the New England Cremation Society in 1895, recalling the first crematory in an early parish of his, "Cremation was considered to be a revival of Paganism. And anyhow, Pagan or not, it was novel

28

and eccentric and we resented it accordingly."[48] The medieval world had been accustomed to Galen's anatomy, based on the structures of animals, so that Pope Leo X (1519) denied Leonardo da Vinci the right to study anatomy in a Roman hospital because he had practiced dissection upon human beings.[49]

The struggle to establish the morality of anesthesia illustrates the reactionary effects of the cake of custom. (A pilgrimage spot for students of ethics and medical care is the Ether Room in the dome of the Massachusetts General Hospital, where anesthesia was first used in New England experimentally[50] and where it received its name from the scholarly Dr. Oliver Wendell Holmes on October 16, 1846.) The use of anesthetics was resisted, here in America and abroad, for a long time. Surgeons who proposed or tried its use were vilified, because it was new and therefore strange, therefore fearful, therefore wrong. Besides, "it might be abused"! *Xenophobia* is the thing that gives customary morality its force. As usual, in the issue over anesthesia, customary morality found an ally in theocratic morality. Many are the uses of religion, and there are always those who have the answer to every moral question that arises merely by consulting an oracle, or maybe a crystal ball, a medium, perchance a high priest or (in a Fundamentalist way) a "book of the words," the Bible. Many Protestant and Catholic clergy alike inveighed against anesthesia, especially when it was employed to ease childbirth. These reverend gentlemen, holding true to their theocratic habits of mind and spirit, appealed to their revealed moral rules, including the claim that suffering was a God-imparted part of life and of the creation, that Job said there was no escape from it, that the Cross taught its indispensable role in salvation,

---

[48] *Reverent Care of the Dead*, addresses by Dr. John Homans, 2nd, and the Rev. George Hodges, D.D., Boston, 1895.

[49] Stern, *op.cit.*, p. 178.

[50] It was first used in Georgia in 1842.

and that anesthesia was therefore "contrary to religion and the express commands of scripture." As evidence that God intended painful childbirth, it was argued that it was a consequence of the Fall and an expiation of original sin. They quoted Genesis 3:16, "Unto the woman he said, I will greatly multiply thy sorrow and thy conception; in sorrow thou shalt bring forth thy children."

But there were also exponents of the third kind of morality, the rational or reflective kind. In 1847, a year following the experiment carried out successfully in the Ether Room, Dr. James Y. Simpson, professor of obstetrics at Glasgow, published a paper entitled *Answer to the Religious Objections Against the Employment of Anesthetic Agents in Midwifery and Surgery*. In addition to the commonsense morality of mercy, and of concern for self-possession rather than demoralizing and disorganizing pain, he had a *coup de grâce* for the Biblicists. He gave them some of their own "medicine" from Genesis, this time 2:21: "And the Lord *caused a deep sleep* to fall upon Adam, and he slept: and he took one of his ribs, and closed up the flesh instead thereof." This, by the same species of logic and authority, made God the first surgical anesthetist, and satisfied the canons of Fundamentalist morality as well as the canons of reason![51]

One other example of religious obstructionism might be mentioned. In this case it was based upon prudery more than upon any theological ground. One hundred years ago there was in America a fierce and morally righteous resistance to the practice of gynecology by male physicians. This, be it noted, was an attitude of puritanical sentiment at almost complete odds with the Christian tradition in Europe. One George Gregory led the attack, taking his text from *Godey's Lady Book*, in the claim that "there are few self-evident propositions," and one of them is that "female physicians are

[51] See the full account in H. H. Haggard, *Devils, Drugs and Doctors*, New York, 1929, p. 100ff.

the proper attendants of their own sex in the hour of sorrow." Using candid plates from *Magrier's Midwifery Illustrated*, he published a book in which this Biblical argument (correct enough in itself) was used: "The Bible repeatedly speaks of women assisting at births, but nowhere in the sacred records, extending over a period of thousands of years, is it intimated that man ever rendered such unnatural services; while it expressly said that 'God dealt well with the midwives.' "[52] (The quotation about midwives is from the preface to the Moses story, Exodus 1:20.) In another pamphlet, *Letters to Ladies, in favor of Female Physicians for their Own Sex* (Boston, 1850), Gregory complained of male attendance at births by asking, "What is it but a system of legalized prostitution? Thus the medical profession is doing more to undermine public virtue than all the ministers of the gospel, and the moral reform societies, can do to preserve it." A clergyman told him that when his wife, "young and acutely sensitive," was confined, she found that the doctor's examination "was more than her philosophy could bear." The emotional maturity of a scientific era, and increasing experience with its medical benefits, appear to have shown that our "philosophies" can bear a heavier load than prurience would ever assume.

We must at all times acknowledge the difference between moral insight and moral power. Neither of these things is a fixed quantity, in any of us. How do we know what is right? And how do we find the power, the strength of will, to *do* it? It seems that in any reasonable and humble view of the matter we can say two things, and say them confidently. One is that we gain our knowledge of right and wrong gradually, from year to year as individuals, and from genera-

[52] *Medical Morals, Illustrated with Plates and Extracts from Medical Works, designed to show the pernicious social and moral influence of the present system of medical practice, and the importance of establishing female medical colleges, and educating and employing female physicians for their own sex.* New York, 1852, pub. by the author. 48 pp.

tion to generation as a community. Our understanding is not "born full-fledged from the brain of Jove," or graven once for all on stone tablets of law. Moral knowledge (or conscience) is a matter of growth, an increase in human capacity. The other thing is that our power or ability to "do the good and hate the evil" is by no means a mere matter of automatic increase, or even of an over-all increase or, in many cases, of any increase at all. To trust, as surely we must, in reflective morality is *not* to make any claim for human self-sufficiency, or to accept a boot-strap theory of moral performance. Although this latter point, directed mainly to humanistic ethics, raises religious questions of a kind which are not within our immediate purview, no valid part of our discussion will fall afoul of the *believing* claim that a power greater than our own is the surest source of our ability to do the good which we would, and to reject the evil which we would not. Christian men call it "grace." And just as moral knowledge is a matter of growth, an increase in a human capacity, so moral power is a matter of grace, an increase in the love of God.

In a very remarkable and heart-warming book of lectures, published in 1929, a symposium called *Physician and Patient: Personal Care*, there is a striking example of the moral insights and sensitivity of medical practitioners.[53] Dr. Lawrence K. Lunt contributed an essay on "Human Nature and its Reaction to Suffering," in which he pointed out, on the basis of long clinical and practical experience, that there are four ways by which we may respond to disease and suffering. We can close this chapter by reciting them, with examples and comments of our own added.

The lowest kind of response, he said, is a reflex action. It has (we should observe) no knowledge in it, no freedom, no personal choice or responsibility. There is no moral quality to the foot's swing when the hammer hits the knee in a

[53] Ed. by L. Eugene Emerson, M.D., Cambridge, 1929.

test for *locomotor ataxia*. Only slightly more complex, and still not one of moral quality since it lacks the elements of rational deliberation and choice, Dr. Lunt suggested an instinctive response as the second kind. We see it, of course, in the dog who chews grass instead of meat, like a cow, when his stomach is off. The third kind of response in the scale of moral quality is the intelligent one. This has *at least one* of the two elements postulated in all moral or human acts; it employs knowledge. It is better, therefore, than blind obedience, which is never truly moral because it is blind, no matter whether the obedience is paid to a custom or a state or a god.

Yet, morally weighed, what Dr. Lunt called the moral response (the fourth one) is the necessary ideal and goal of the ethics of medical care. Those who meet disease and suffering with true personal knowledge of their condition, like the diabetic patient who administers his own shots with the doctor's guidance, those who assume personal responsibility for treatment, who exercise the personal freedom to choose the medical course and care to be rendered—such people are moral beings. Without their freedom to choose and their right to know the truth, patients are only puppets. And there is no moral quality in a Punch and Judy show; at least there is none in Punch or Judy! It was not because we are only automatons or pawns in the flux of nature ("red in tooth and claw") that Hamlet marvelled, "What a piece of work man is!"

CHAPTER TWO

MEDICAL DIAGNOSIS:
OUR RIGHT TO KNOW THE TRUTH

The Truth Can Hurt

A GENTLEMAN," said Dr. John M. Birnie in the *New England Journal of Medicine*, "is one who has more regard for the rights of others than for his own feelings, and for the feelings of others than for his own rights."[1] Disraeli, bemused by the troublesome problem of truth-telling, put it this way: "A gentleman is one who knows when to tell the truth, and when not to." His diplomatic impulses served him better than the cynic's who observed that "a gentleman is one who never unintentionally hurts the feelings of others." But Dr. Birnie meant, presumably, that the gentle person is one who avoids saying anything that *needlessly* hurts a person's feelings.

The issue over truth-telling in medical diagnosis and advice raises the question, therefore, whether doctors can be "gentlemen" and at the same time meet their obligations to the patients under their care. What, to be quite to the point about it, is the duty of the physician in sharing his diagnosis and prognosis? Is he under any obligation morally to reveal his findings to his patient, even if it hurts to know them? Has the patient, in his turn, a right to expect the truth? Or are we to accept the bold claim by Dumas' heroine in *Camille* who declared, "When God said that lying was a sin, he made an exception for doctors, and he gave them permission to lie as many times a day as they saw patients"? It is an old and perennial problem, giving cause in every age to complaints against doctors as masters of equivocation, complaints sometimes made with great hilarity by a Gregory Glyster.[2] This

[1] 205.1126, "Ethics for the Doctor."
[2] *A Dose for the Doctor; or, the Aesculapian Labyrinth Explored in a Series*

is the kind of question in people's minds which popular interpreters never undertake to clarify.

We have already set forward the premise that moral status (our ethical integrity) depends upon two things at least: first, freedom of choice, and, second, knowledge of the facts and of the courses between which we may choose. In the absence of either or both of these things we are, in the forum of conscience, more like puppets than persons. Lacking freedom[3] and knowledge, we are not responsible; we are not moral agents or personal beings. We have pointed out, furthermore, that mankind is constantly growing and gaining ground both in knowledge of life and health and in human control over them. This is, indeed, the same as saying that the *means* to heightened moral stature are available. The appeal of moral idealism is that we take advantage of every opportunity to grow in wisdom and stature, that we *assume* our responsibility; in short, that we act like human beings. As far as medical care is concerned we can only repeat what we said above: "Without their freedom to choose and their right to know the truth, patients are only puppets. And there is no moral quality in a Punch and Judy show; at least, there is none in Punch or Judy!"

Dr. Birnie's dilemma was a real one. Sometimes the doctor's discoveries are appalling. To whom, then, shall he give his findings? As a gentleman he hates to hurt his patients' feelings, to depress them, or possibly to drive them to despair. When the truth about our health is a bitter pill to swallow, known as yet only to the physician and perhaps not even suspected by those who put themselves in his hands, he will of course have compassionate regard for their

---

of Instructions to Young Physicians, Surgeons, Accouchers, Apothecaries, Druggists and Chymists, Interspersed with a variety of Risible Anecdotes Affecting the Faculty. Inscribed to the College of Wigs, by Gregory Glyster, an old practitioner. London, 1789. In the Warren Collection, Harvard Medical School Library.

[3] By freedom we mean *physical* freedom, what we *can* do; not moral freedom, referring to what we *may* do.

feelings. For this reason—a perfectly understandable one—
Dr. Birnie concluded that "in hopeless cases, it is cruel and
harmful to tell the patient the truth," and even if the doctor
tells some member of the family it will be necessary for both
"to lie like gentlemen."[4] It is a hoary old problem of conscience in medical care. For our purposes we may attempt
to explore it by posing two questions between which to
shuttle back and forth. They are really obverse sides of the
same coin, but they represent two distinguishable issues involved. First, has the patient a *right* to know the truth about
himself? Next, has the doctor an *obligation* to tell it? Most
of us upon occasion are patients, but only a few are physicians. The discussion, therefore, will naturally and properly
tend to emphasize the first viewpoint and its question,
namely, the *patient's right*.

If the doctor is thus obliged to tell the truth, what difference would it make if the patient is not sure he wants to
know it, or if he actually does not want to know it? This
question raises a matter of almost crucial importance for
psychotherapy, and even for the less pathological areas of
clinical counselling. And (most difficult of all) what if the
doctor cannot know whether the patient wants to know?
Is there a valid principle of therapeutic reservation when it
comes to truth-telling in medical diagnosis? Very good
reason would have to be found—better, at least than has ever
been brought forward—to justify us in avoiding the answer
that follows from the premise that our moral stature is proportionate to our responsibility and that we cannot act responsibly without the fullest possible knowledge. The patient
has a right to know the truth. We are morally obligated to
pay others the rights due them. Therefore a doctor is obligated to tell the truth to his patient. He *owes* the patient the
truth as fully and as honestly as he owes him his skill and
care and technical powers.

[4] Birnie, *op.cit.*, same place.

We have already expressed the view that "a person-centered approach to illness is superior to the problem-centered approach." To support it we quoted Dr. Francis Peabody's thesis that "one of the essential qualities of the clinician is interest in humanity, for the secret of the care of the patient is caring *for* the patient."[5] What does it mean to care *for* somebody? The mere business of taking care *of* a person may be entirely a matter of efficiency, and quite impersonal, as many of us have discovered by watching the ministrations of a very young or very bored nurse (or waiter, clerk in a store, barber, or dentist). Caring *for* a person, on the other hand, is a decidedly moral relationship. The phrase "care for" has even come in popular speech to mean love or highly affectionate regard. It means, of course, that we have a care, a sense of concern. A man is said to care for his wife, and that means vastly more than providing for her physical needs; it means a lot more than offering fuel, shelter, food, and clothing. It means, indeed, that he has an attitude of respect and solicitude towards her in all things. So should the doctor's attitude be toward his patient. The sufferer is not just a case of pneumonia or pyloric stenosis or peptic ulcer; the patient is a person, with feelings of hope or despair, of purpose or defeat, of loneliness or fraternity. The patient is not a problem; he is a person with a problem.

From the point of view of morality, we might look at this question as it would be seen by Martin Buber, philosopher at the University of Jerusalem.[6] There is, as Buber points out, a radical difference in a man's attitude to other men and his attitude to things. In the one case we are related to other persons, like ourselves, to another subject, a *thou*. In the other case we are related to objects, to things, to *its*. These are the two attitudes with which we relate ourselves to what

---

[5] See ch. 1, n. 13.

[6] *I and Thou*, trans. by R. G. Smith, Edinburgh, 1937. Cf. also by the same author, *Between Man and Man*, New York, 1948, pp. 1-80, 118-205.

is other than ourselves. A doctor's patient is a person, a *thou*, someone with an integrity and a moral quality of his own. Relationship to persons is a moral experience because persons are responsible (they can *respond*). Unlike things, they can say "yes" or "no." They have rights, especially the right to say "yes" or "no" in response (in being responsible), the right to self-determination, the right to be themselves, to choose; in short, to be a *thou* and not an *it*, a subject and not an object.[7]

The ethical importance of this distinction is plain enough. We have reasoned thus far that the moral stature of men and women is directly proportionate to the freedom they enjoy, that their freedom to choose is, in its turn, proportionate to the control they have gained over their alternatives of action and to *the knowledge they possess of the alternatives open to them*. If a patient is simply an object of medical treatment, who submits without any knowledge of his condition and its prognosis, that patient has ceased to be a *thou*, has become an *it*. He is being manipulated as a thing, not met and accredited as a person. He has lost his place in the forum of conscience; he is deprived of responsibility and therefore of moral status. This is the ethical implication of the belief that physicians ought to serve according to the demands of a person-centered rather than of a problem-centered approach to the patient's suffering.[8] Something of this philosophy of practice is surely working like a leaven in the medical schools and in the profession itself. It was a common feature of the work of the old country doctor, even though his role has been somewhat romantically colored from time to time. When medical technology and urbanism had not yet outmoded the practice of medicine out of a little

[7] This dialogical thesis in one of its dimensions is a refreshing reformulation of Kant's old axiom: so act as to use humanity, both in your own person and in others, always as an end and never as a means.

[8] The doctor must do both things, however, for all the sympathy in the world will not compensate for a wrong diagnosis.

black bag, it was psychologically easier to maintain a strong personal factor in the physician-patient relationship. The dangers of specialism, in this regard, have stimulated efforts to recover the human values of general practice, as we may see in the experiments of the Peter Bent Brigham Hospital and the Harvard Medical School in teaching "integrated medicine." As Dr. Henry M. Fox, director of the unit, says: "The pendulum which has swung so far from the personal interest of the country doctor to the more detached attitude of the specialist is now swinging back to a halfway mark maintaining the good features of each."[9] In public reports of this study it is significant that one of its features receiving special attention is an effort to discover whether the patient "needs more information to relieve his worries or his wonderment about what is going on."[10]

"What Is Truth?"

To say, however, that the doctor owes the truth to his patient does not altogether cover the ground of conscience involved. First of all, we ought to recognize that this right to know the truth does not apply to all truths. There are secrets of others, for example, to which few if any of us have any right at all. Furthermore, the classic question put by Pilate to Jesus, "What is truth?" can be applied to the problem of medical diagnosis and truth-telling.[11] As Pilate's question seems to have been intended to suggest, none of us has perfect knowledge; also, the human intelligence with which we try to make sense of what knowledge we have is not infallible. Given a doctor's willingness and desire to respect the patient's right to know the truth, how shall he convey it? How can he be *sure*? In the tradition of ethics and moral theology in Western Christendom it has generally been said that truth is of two kinds, logical truth and moral

[9] *Boston Sunday Herald*, July 15, 1951.
[10] *Ibid.*   [11] John 18:38.

truth. This distinction appears to have considerable bearing upon the problem of truth-telling as between physician and patient. Logical truth (or accuracy) is the correspondence of outward or verbal expressions to or with the matter which is the subject of the expression. Moral truth (or veracity) is the correspondence of the outward expression given to our thought, with the thought itself. Accuracy, in other words, is telling the truth as it actually is, at least as far as our knowledge of it goes; veracity is telling the truth honestly and not withholding or changing or obscuring a part of what we believe to be true.

When it comes to telling the truth, we can never be sure that we know it, nor can we always be sure that we convey it as we *do* know it or believe it to be. Our modern sociology of knowledge, and psychology with its new understanding of the subtleties of communication and the role of the unconscious, have humbled us a great deal about our capacity either to grasp or to convey the truth. But these considerations are only cautionary; they have to do only with the negative defects of truth, due to human limitations, not with positive injuries to the truth, due to willful distortion and suppression. Problems of morality or of conscience in connection with truth-telling arise only in the case of moral truth (veracity), not with logical truth (accuracy).

It is presumed that inaccuracy or error, in the case of medical advice or in any other area, is unintentional and therefore by definition entirely outside the forum of conscience. In short, as far as morality is concerned (although not so far as science is concerned) what is at stake in telling the truth is, precisely, honesty. Dr. John Homans once protested, "There can be no universal rule to tell the brutal truth. And the first and best reason for not telling the truth is the impossibility of being certain what the truth is."[12] But this admitted fact is too often a red herring, drawn across the

[12] *The Care of the Patient from the Surgeon's Standpoint*, Boston, 1934.

trail to confuse conscience, since it bears only upon the problem of accuracy, not upon the problem of honesty. Indeed, a part of the truth which the doctor owes the patient is just that: that the doctor cannot be absolutely correct. After all, doctors, like their patients, have to be prepared to meet frustration through knowledge. Their very science often gives them an insight into bitter realities which would leave the primitive medicine-man, who could not know, reasonably hopeful. To take refuge in finitude to avoid reality is only a sophisticated form of escapism, when it is used as an excuse for departing from honesty. No: the question before us really is: *are we obliged to tell the truth as we see it according to our best knowledge?* For this very reason it is a matter of simple justice that the law does not require a physician to be responsible for errors in judgment, or to possess any unusual skill beyond the average. This is the principle of law under which every issue of professional responsibility is adjudicated. Indefectibility of the person—whether in knowledge, skill, or strength—is assumed to be out of the question. Therefore, to deny the obligation of truth-telling by pointing to human limitations is neither here nor there.

St. Augustine said a lie is always and necessarily sinful.[13] Thomas Aquinas in the Middle Ages said, "A lie has the character of sinfulness, not only from the damage done to a neighbor, but also from its own inordinateness. . . . And therefore [he concludes] it is not lawful to tell a lie to deliver another from any danger whatever."[14] It is true that St. Thomas went on to say, "It is lawful, however, to hide the truth prudently under some dissimulation, as Augustine says." But this reference to St. Augustine's opinion (in *De mendacio*, 2) that we are permitted to tell an obvious, joking fib, deliberately shown to be such by one's tone of voice and manner, does not alter the principle at all. For such lying

[13] *Enchiridion*, 18; *De mendacio*, 6.21.
[14] *Summa theologica*, ii.-ii.110.3ff.

is legitimate since, after all, a lie which advertises itself as such is no longer really a lie. Or, again, a lie which is of the nature of evident fiction is not a real falsehood. Also, there are times when, as Jeremy Taylor put it in the seventeenth century, "we may lie to children and idiots." He tells of how one Hercules of Saxonia, a medical practitioner, saved the life of a madman who imagined himself to be Elijah and refused to take food, by sending him a "fellow dressed like an angel" with the command to rise and eat.[15] Here, in this patient, was a lack of moral capacity or responsibility. Such sufferers are, in this respect, like children who are irresponsible through inexperience, and like idiots who lack moral capacity through mental deficiency. They are not morally responsible agents. But adults, as Taylor himself insisted, *are* persons of responsibility. Yet he explains without protest that in his day "to lie like a physician" was a complimentary remark.[16] It is also interesting, in this connection, to see how the author of *Holy Living* and *Holy Dying* was entirely ready to permit a doctor to lie to his patient, even when dying, whereas he would have been morally outraged had a *priest* lied to the same patient! The sacrament of extreme unction and last Confessions are practices whereby ministers of religion demonstrate that *they* do not scruple to let the dying or the seriously ill know the real situation. Here again is that curious and persistent assumption (working like an ethical termite) that the doctor is dealing with a body, a physical *thing*, and that he therefore has no moral obligation to the patient's personality and spiritual integrity. It assumes, at least, that the doctor has none compared to the obligations of a priest or pastor on the spiritual level. But from any view except the crudest materialism, the physician is just as responsibly related to the patient as a moral subject

---

[15] *Ductor Dubitantium*, iii.2,5; i.5,8, par. 28.
[16] Cf. a parallel discussion in K. E. Kirk, *Conscience and Its Problems*, London, 1927, p. 123.

42

as any priest could be, for the spirit and the body are one.

In our day doctors commonly act according to Taylor's latitude.[17] The indecision and evasion over the nature of a lie, which we all have felt and fought with, is seen in the public words of one practitioner, whom we shall leave unidentified even though his statement was part of a lecture to medical students: "Personally, I can, I think, truthfully say that in a practice of forty years I never, as far as I can remember, found it necessary to tell an outright lie to a patient about his condition. Tactful and skillful explanations with their if's and and's, side issues and suggestions of possibilities, always sufficiently befogged the issue, satisfied the patient, and left my conscience unseared. A sick man is not a well man and what would be injudicious to say to the one is often swallowed with almost a real relish by the other." Here, in these tortuous terms, are all the involutions of our problem!

From the earliest times it has been argued that a lie is not a lie if there is a just cause for it. Among such just causes men have included self-defense, military necessity, and even zeal for God's honor! The kindly old Jesuit of the *Provincial Letters* was no purely modern phenomenon. Pious frauds, miracle stories, false decretals, bogus relics, and the like are an early and common story. Cardinal Newman felt that the majority of church moralists had by their defense of falsehood *per causa justa* further impaired the Christian's sense of truth.[18] Theologians argued that since faith need not be kept with a tyrant or a robber, it is still less to be kept with a heretic who kills the soul. Gregory of

---

[17] A leading Catholic moralist says, "A deplorable pagan custom is in vogue among many doctors today—the custom of deceiving their patients about their condition so effectively that they slip out of life without realizing that they are dying." F. J. Connell, *Morals in Politics and Professions*, Westminster, Md., 1946, p. 122.

[18] *Apologia pro vita sua*, New York, 1865, 291ff., esp. p. 300; on the principle of *Corruptio optimi est pessima* he reproves the amphibilogia of the casuists and their economy of truth.

Nyssa, Origen, and most of the later Fathers even argued that God himself used deceit in dealing with his enemy the Devil. He did so, they said, by offering him Christ's soul in exchange for the souls of sinful men, knowing all the time that the Devil could not *keep* the ransom paid him, since the soul of Christ was sinless and would torture the Devil unbearably. Some Christians in the past have tried to defend the lies recorded in the Bible. Since the Bible gives a more or less outright condemnation of lying in certain passages, these attempts have usually been made to prove that the lies were not really lies at all, and thus that they are conformable to the theory that there is no internal contradiction in Holy Writ. They have written some marvellous commentaries on Rahab's lie, and that of the midwives in Egypt; on Jehu's sacrilegious Baal-worship in order to slaughter the Baal-worshipers; on David's trickeries; Jacob's deception of Isaac; Abraham's lie about Sarah and hers to the angel. The opinion condemning lying, quoted above from St. Augustine, was written as part of an answer to St. Jerome's attempt to explain away the statement in Galatians 2:11 that two saintly apostles disagreed and struggled against each other over the question of eating with Gentiles. Paul accuses Peter of being a sycophant and a weathercock, but this contradicts the account in Acts of a harmonious meeting of the apostolic council. St. Jerome, following Origen's lead, had argued that Peter engaged in one deliberate lie (he only pretended to reject the company of Gentiles), and Paul in two (he only pretended to condemn Peter, and his account to the Galatians was a falsehood to avoid annoying the Gentiles).[19] All of these were perpetrated in order to eliminate the Jewish restrictions on Christian eating habits. A contradiction in the Scriptures was looked upon as far more undesirable than a reputation for lying in the apostles whose activities they recorded.

[19] Cf. A. Harnack, *History of Dogma*, II, 367, n. 1.

Actually, the Bible has no clear and consistent teaching on the question of falsehood explicitly, even though the spirit of the Wisdom literature in the Old Testament (especially Proverbs) and a couple of Pauline verses are clearly against it. Lying was a besetting sin from Jacob onwards. In the Commandments it is perjury which is forbidden, as we can see in the penalties provided in Deuteronomy 19:51, and calumny as well, to judge by Exodus 23:1. The passage in Leviticus 19:11, "Ye shall not steal, neither deal falsely, neither lie one to another," has to do with contracts and fair dealing in exchange matters. There is no outright condemnation of lying in the Beatitudes nor in the Sermon on the Mount, although the whole ethos of the Gospel is alien to lying. In the Fourth Gospel, the saying, "Ye shall know the truth, and the truth shall make you free" (8:32) refers to a particular truth about God. Paul establishes honesty as a sectarian or brotherhood virtue in Colossians 3:9: "Lie not to one another, seeing that you have put off the old man and his deeds." The story of Ananias and Sapphira (Acts 5:1-6) falls into this latter class. There *may* be a broader application in mind when St. Paul says, Ephesians 4:25, "Wherefore putting away lying, speak every man truth with his neighbor; for we are members one of another." In any case, deception has consistently been held (in the abstract) to be a fault against virtue, and no moralist has ever attempted to defend it *in principle*.

Is Ignorance Bliss?

There are many ways by which a physician can deceive his patient, either by misrepresenting the facts as he sees them or by withholding them. Our opinion is that in either case such deceptions are morally speaking unlawful, being acts of theft because they keep from the patient what is rightfully his (the truth about himself), or acts of injustice because they deny to another what is his due as a free and responsible person. The most dramatic case of conscience in medical diagnosis and truth-telling has to do, of course, with the patient who is found to be the victim of a possibly or probably fatal disease, or one for whom no hope at all can be held out. In medical practice, as a matter of fact, there are many other diagnoses that entail sadness equal to or greater than the sadness that is caused by the malignant neoplasms; there are such conditions as brain damage in babies, leading to spastic paralysis, cardio-vascular diseases with poor prognosis, and the like. Yet even in terminal diseases the reaction of patients to the truth is varied and unpredictable. Dr. Fred C. Shattuck relates that one cancer patient, a cheerful businessman, never smiled again after he was told the truth, apparently crushed in spirit. But another patient, fretful and troublesome, who complained constantly at the discomfort, pulled himself together and showed great courage and moral vigor to the last.[20] Experienced pastors can tell of episodes wherein their own faith has been deepened by the faith and assurance and joy with which terminal patients faced death, sometimes over a long period, and in some cases *not until* they were made fully aware of the truth. But fear of the truth is very strong in many people, including physicians, and this fear accounts for the fact that from ancient to modern times no universal or local code of medical ethics has ever attempted to regulate the doctor's conscience in matters of truth-telling. The first code on the tablets of Hammurabi, 2080 B.C., said nothing about it; the confessors' manuals of the Middle Ages dealing with the rules of shriving surgeons and leechers said nothing; the latest code of the American Medical Association, by its silence or equivocation, leaves the whole thing up to the individual practitioner.

Suppose we turn for a moment to the opinion set forth by Dr. Richard C. Cabot, who was for so many years a physician and teacher at the Massachusetts General Hospital. As Pro-

[20] "Medical Ethics," address at Western Reserve College, Apr. 25, 1908.

fessor of Social Ethics in Harvard University and Lecturer in Pastoral Care at Andover-Newton Theological School and at the Episcopal Theological School, Dr. Cabot followed his art and his conscience wherever they took him, into hospitals, laboratories, social agencies (he was President of the National Conference of Social Work), and into the labyrinth of morals. In the last of his books to be published (*Honesty*, in 1939) he included an enlightening chapter on "Honesty and Dishonesty in Medicine." After a long life of medical service and the most constant moral concern, he wrote: "As a young physician I tried the usual system of benevolent lying from 1893 to 1902. About that time a bitter experience convinced me that I could not be an amateur liar, an occasional, philanthropic liar in medicine or in any part of life. I swore off and have been on the water wagon of medical honesty ever since."[21]

In another work, written some years earlier (*The Meaning of Right and Wrong*), Dr. Cabot put the matter along these lines: "How can we ever be sure where a conscientious liar will draw the line? It appears to me, therefore, that the doctrine that it is sometimes right to lie can never be effectively asserted. For our hearers take notice, and so make ineffective our subsequent attempts to lie. I recall a sick man who ordered his physician never to tell him the truth in case he should be seriously ill. Picture the state of that sick man's mind when later he hears his physician's reassurances. 'Perhaps he really doesn't consider this sickness a serious one. Then he will be telling me the truth!' How can the sick man know? If he asks the doctor whether he considers the disease serious and gets a negative answer, how is he to interpret that answer? If the doctor did consider the disease serious he would also have to say 'No.' His words have become mere wind. No one can interpret them. His reassuring

[21] *Op.cit.*, pp. 134-156.

manner, his smiles, his cheering tones may be true or they may be lies. Who can say?

"Suppose the disease comes to a point which demands operation. But to mention operation is to let the patient know that his trouble is serious, and that is forbidden. Shall the doctor therefore let the operation go and let the patient get worse? Whatever he does or says his patient has grounds for fearing the worst. No reassurance can be taken at its face value. The most trifling ailment must be suspect; good news may always mean bad.

"Here then is a self-enforcing moral law. 'Thou shalt not confess to a belief in occasional lies.' "[22]

Dr. Cabot then goes on to point out that if you *do not* admit that you tell conscientious lies, you make yourself an unconscientious liar. "For the very conscientiousness of conscientious lies depends on their being known to be exceptions to the rule. No one can be a universal conscientious liar." He was, in his own way, reaching the view put long ago in an old German proverb, *Wer einmal lügt dem glaubt man nicht, und wenn er auch die Warheit spricht* (he who once lies is never believed, even when he is telling the truth).[23]

A good example of the dilemma here is to be found in the newspapers of February 1923. The prize fighter J. J. Corbett had died of cancer, and *The New York Times* ran the story with this headline: "Ex-Champion Succumbs Here to Cancer. He Believed He Had Heart Disease." Such was the conscientious lie with which Gentlemen Jim's doctor had let him live out his last days. However, other doctors soon began violently to protest the open publication of the deception in a news story, one physician complaining to the editor that several of his own patients with heart diseases were wild with fear that they too really had cancer of the liver. G. K. Chesterton in his *Life of Browning* said, "Mrs.

[22] New York, 1933, pp. 167-168.
[23] Cf. a supporting opinion by Edith M. Stern, *McCall's Magazine*, Aug. 1951.

Browning was surrounded by that most poisonous and degrading of all atmospheres, a medical atmosphere."[24] We can be thankful that great strides have been made in the past century towards humanizing the sick room and the hospital, but there will always be an element of degradation in it as long as sensitive and self-respecting patients have reason to suspect that they are being lied to by their medical servants, no matter how kindly the motives may be. Truth-telling is essential to any personal, thou-thou, relationship; just as essential as love, *agápe*, solicitude. The two go together, trust and truth; they require and presuppose each other. Paul's phrase (Ephesians 4:15), "speaking the truth in love," applies not only to our growth in Christ but to our growth in all relationships higher than *I-it*. On a broader scale in the body politic, it is vital to our whole democratic ideal. Government of, by, and for the people is only a myth unless it adheres to the principle that human beings act and respond on the basis of what they know, not on what is concealed from them. There is no responsibility once knowledge is denied or subject to cheating.

There is inescapably a subversive result of occasional lying. It makes no real difference whether it is perpetrated by a direct commission of an untruth, or indirectly through the omission of a truth. Lying troubles the waters of human relations and takes away the one element of mutual trust without which medical practice becomes a manipulation of bodies rather than the care of and for persons. The assumption made by the physician, when he has the *presumption* to withhold the truth, is that the patient is really no longer an adult, but rather either a child or an idiot, more an *it* than a *thou*. In this connection we should note that medical experience by no means lends support to the idea that telling the patient ominous truths will aggravate a serious condition. Some

---

[24] Quoted by R. C. Cabot, *Psychotherapy and Its Relation to Religion*, New York, 1908.

years ago the Division of Cancer in the Massachusetts Department of Public Health issued a bulletin in which it was said, "The fallacious argument [that lies are necessary] may be answered as follows. . . . [We find that] those physicians and hospitals making a practice of telling the patients frankly when they have the disease, report only the fullest cooperation of the patient in his treatment. But the physician who lies to his patient denies him a chance to show his common sense and helps him one step nearer to the undertaker."[25]

Dr. Cabot, as we have seen, put forward a number of good reasons for truth-telling in medical care. In much of what he had to say he was answering a statement by Dr. Joseph Collins, who had defended medical falsehoods in *Harper's Magazine* for August 1927 in an article entitled "Should Doctors Tell the Truth?" Dr. Cabot pointed out, among other things, that without the truth patients will often object to decisive and costly forms of treatment, surgical or otherwise, since their urgency will not be apparent while the cost will be. If the patient is not told of approaching death, or at least of its grave possibility, he may fail to make proper preparation for his death in wills and testaments, or in reparations and restorations of one kind or another, or in reconciliations with God and/or men. Respect for the *rights* of a man whose time is running out is the real meaning of that famous petition in the Anglican litany: "From lightning and tempest . . . [plus a long list of other calamities] and from *sudden death*, good Lord, deliver me." It is not death itself that is the calamity, but its sudden coming.[26] Sudden death is the extreme fatality, and (as we have already observed) fatality is the denial and negation of morality. In the ethical perspective, fatality is nothing more nor less

---

[25] *Cancer Clinic Bulletin*, No. 41, Dec. 1936.

[26] I am indebted to a friend, a Roman Catholic moralist, who has pointed out to me that the Roman "Litany of the Saints" is even more explicit: "a subitanea et improvisa morte" (from a sudden and *unprovided* death).

than willy-nilly helplessness, being pushed around by circumstances in ignorance.

Furthermore, only a little experience with doctors, patients' families, and ministers of religion as they deal with terminal diseases or some other condition threatening death or helplessness is enough to show that a great deal of the time their evasion of the plain truth is a protective mechanism for themselves, a rationalization of their own embarrassment and dis-ease. Much of our human behavior, even among doctors, is aimed at satisfying our own needs, emotional and otherwise, not the needs of others. It is a fact to be faced that reservation or corruption of the truth is not always based on a genuine and maturely weighed decision that the patient "is just as well off if he (or she) doesn't know." Fear, we repeat, leads to lies. Fear and lies tend to require and presuppose each other, as do love and truth. Perhaps we need not feel so threatened emotionally by the truth. Dr. Walter Alvarez of the Mayo Clinic says, "often it is the relatives who have fear and mental pain. . . . In forty-odd years of practice I cannot remember anyone's committing suicide because I told him the hopeless truth. Instead hundreds of persons thanked me from their hearts and told me I had relieved their minds." Who are we to choose ignorance for others? We *have* to make the choice for animals, because they are animals, incapable of receiving or making creative use of such knowledge. But *ought* we to make it for men?

These considerations apply with just as much force to illnesses of the kind that are far from fatal. Even in imaginary illnesses of a neurasthenic nature, the common practice of the medical lie called "placebo" or the bread pill, the "pink water" or the "water subcut" (a pretended hypodermic), can be shown to undermine a truly moral relationship between physician and patient. A false pill of sugar, or something of the sort to deceive the patient into thinking he receives treatment or medication, is a self-defeating practice. In the first place, it *is* a deception, however well meant. In the second place, it is amazing how few good liars (to use a curious and contradictory phrase) there are, especially in such intimate relationships as illness and medical care. A good many doctors would be well advised, in the light of what we know nowadays about the dynamics of personal relationships, to rely instead, for supportive therapy and encouragement, upon a confident and genuine empathy. In the third place, these practices encourage the idea among neurotic patients that drugs will cure most ailments, and thus serve to extend the patent-medicine evil.

It may be pointed out, of course, that psychiatrists *on principle* do not in all cases share their diagnoses with the patient. Sometimes ignorance is bliss in correcting mental and emotional disorders. It might be claimed that something of the same therapeutic principle may apply to the general practitioner in his work. But for one thing we can answer that the cases are not parallel, inasmuch as the psychiatrist withholds his knowledge precisely because he may prevent the patient's recovery by revealing it, at least if he does so too soon. It is by no means evident that the same is true if the truth has to do with a pink pill for an imaginary illness, or with a diagnosis of cancer disguised to the patient as a tumor, or a heart disease camouflaged as overweight or indigestion. And in any case, the psychiatrist's ministrations are not even relevant in cases where imminent death or its probability is a chief reality factor, or in cases of primarily physical pathology, surgery, and the like.

There is no good reason, merely out of rigid adherence to abstract principle, to be hard or brutally logical about the morality of truth-telling in illness and dying. On the other hand it seems fair to say that the right of the patient to know the truth is clear on moral grounds, and this is true whether or not our ultimate sanction for loyalty to truth and to personal rights is religious. Our argument would lose none of its force by accepting the non-doctrinaire view reported in *The Journal of the American Medical Association*: "Some feel that a humanistic philosophy affords an adequate basis; some find in the teachings of Christ the highest concept of the meaning of a life of service."[27] Any sensitive person can sympathize with Dr. Alfred Worcester, who showed in the following plaintive remark that he recognized his duty to tell the truth yet disliked it: "Devotion to the truth does not always require the physician to voice his fears or tell his patient all he knows. But, after he had decided that the process of dying has actually begun, only in exceptional circumstances would a physician be justified in keeping to himself his opinion. In such cases his only question should be whether to tell the patient or the family, and, when both are to be told, which to tell first."[28] Dr. Worcester's surrender to conscience is questionable only insofar as, like St. Paul, who "kicked against the pricks," he tried to transfer his debt to his patient by farming it out to the family as middlemen or brokers.

The Medical Code on Lying

The A.M.A. *Code of Ethics*, 1940, says (in Chapter Two): "A physician should give timely notice of dangerous manifestations of the disease to the friends of the patient." Not, we should notice, to the patient himself! The Code goes on to say, still with patent uncertainty, that the doctor should "assure himself that the patient *or* his friends have such knowledge of the patient's condition as will serve the best interests of the patient and his family." It should be obvious that this is assuming much more knowledge of a family's affairs than medical care, as such, would normally provide. And again, how often the family's and the patient's idea

[27] "Factors Influencing Ethical Concepts and Ideals Among Medical Students," 113:1267-1270.
[28] "The Care of the Dying," *Physician and Patient*, Cambridge, 1929, p. 220.

of the best interests at stake are not the same! How often by keeping the patient in ignorance precisely the opposite of what the patient would want has in fact come about, perhaps through a consequent failure to change a will, or to add a codicil, or to make some explanation to a loved one— all of these being things which only the patient could have done had he known the true state of affairs. It is also ironical to observe how often doctors and families are mistaken in supposing that the patient can be fooled by evasion and suppression of the truth. Dr. William H. Robey, in the George Washington Gay lecture of 1936, asserted that "the family is not to be fooled by any dissimulation."[29] Why, then, imagine that the patient is any easier to fool? Patients may sometimes be at a very low ebb and still show an almost preternatural awareness. If any self-possession at all remains, they are still persons with a person's right to know the truth. It is cruel and inhuman to leave them in doubt, suspicious and confused. Furthermore, it is an insult to be babied whether big or little issues are concerned. Dr. Weir Mitchell tells of once sending a colleague to see an old Quaker lady. Next time he saw her she said to him, "Never send that man to see me again. Thee knowest I do not like to have my feelings poulticed."[30]

A strange inconsistency is also to be found in the *Code of Ethics*. Following the equivocation we have already noted, it declares (Chapter Three, article three, section two) that in cases of medical consultation "all the physicians interested in the case should be frank and candid with the patient and his family." It is not at all clear why a medical consultant should thus be directly charged to be candid with the patient when the physician in charge is not. Yet even here the Code qualifies itself by remarking at another point that the consultant should "state the result of his study to the patient *or*

[29] *New England Journal of Med.*, 205:18, pp. 856-872.
[30] *Ibid.*

his next friend in the presence of the physician in charge." And after all this temporizing about the doctor's obligation to tell the patient the truth, the Code ends with a Golden Rule of medicine, that the physician should "constantly behave towards others as he desires them to deal with him." But can it really be that doctors who practice professional deception would, if the roles were reversed, want to be coddled or deceived? If this is actually the moral standard of those practitioners who deny their patients the truth, then one can only marvel to find so many who are themselves willing, as the Quaker lady expressed it, to have their feeling "poulticed," and willing to be denied knowledge of the most decisive events of their lives, whether it is a fact of health or the final fact of death itself.

The tradition in Western civilization allows for what the law calls "privileged communications" between patient and physician, as between people and pastor. This, indeed, is one of the few priestly aspects of the doctor's role left over from the ancient times. What we tell our doctors and our clergymen is private, personal, our own; and in that sense, secret. Now, as it bears upon truth-telling, the significant thing is that this ethical principle of the professional secret rests upon the conviction that knowledge of a person's private life gained in the course of professional services is a *trust,* the stewardly possession by a professional servant of what belongs to another. The secrets of the confessional box and pastor's study, and of the consulting room and clinic, *belong* to the person served, not to the priest or to the physician. They therefore have no *right* to pass them on to others *without the owner's consent.* By the nature of his office the priest has only that knowledge of a penitent's life which is already known to the penitent and shared by him with the priest. In the case of medicine, however, the physician, the diagnostician, gains knowledge of the patient which (in the nature of the case) the patient does not yet have. But it is still the patient's knowledge and information; it is his life and health which are at stake. The patient has "opened his books" to the doctor on the reasonable assumption that what is found there will be turned over to him, just as a business firm has a right to expect no deception or suppression from an auditor. In spite of all this, some doctors assume the god-like power to ignore the propriety or proper ownership of the secret. On their own behalf they will insist upon the rule of privileged communication, expressing righteous indignation when others attempt to pry or extort information from them; at the same time, however, what they have refused others as not rightfully theirs to give, they will also deny to the patient himself, the rightful owner! Or, with a strange further confusion of ethical reasoning, they will deny the patient the truth which belongs to him, and then proceed to give it to his family or friends, regardless of the principle of professional secrecy.

Before we leave this subject of privileged communications, there is one more related problem of conscience to be faced. Must a doctor remain silent because of professional secrecy if a young man he is treating for syphilis proposes to marry a girl who, according to the doctor's best belief, is ignorant of the fact? This is only an example, although a shocking one, of the general question whether professional confidences may be violated when the interests of "an innocent third party" are at stake. If we use the analogy of property rights again, as we have above in relation to the right of patients to know the truth about themselves, it seems fairly clear that in such a case doctors should "break the seal." Just as in property law and principle there is a rule of eminent domain, in which is expressed the conscience of the community that private property may be expropriated for the sake of a wider welfare of "innocent third parties," so the same qualification of rights, the same expropriation, applies to professional secrets.[31] Even in the most rigorous and exacting moral theology it is recognized that although secrets are obligatory, they can "be modified by the exigencies of public welfare."[32] Apart from secrets of the confessional (*secretum sacramentale, sigillum confessionis*), Catholic moralists allow what the Christian conscience has always provided for, that a legitimate lifting of the rule of secrecy "would be the case, for example, if an innocent man were to suffer serious injury unless a secret were disclosed" in order to prevent it.[33] This has been the position taken by civil courts in the English common law tradition. But surely, to go a step further in the reasoning here, we can question whether there is any good *ethical* ground for making an exception in the case of the seal of confession to a minister. Both the physician and the clergyman should be on the same footing in this regard. The same consideration of *charity* (the welfare of others) would apply to both professional secrets. The priest and his penitent are subject to the ethic of *agápe*, Christian love, which is a disinterested, self-denying love of neighbor. The physician is subject to eminent domain or the public welfare, and although these latter terms are not as idealistic in their connotations as *agápe* or "charity," they have the same force in practice. It would seem almost self-evident that, except for reasons of institutional expedience (such as creating confidence in the inviolability of the confessional "no matter what"), the argument that the *sigillum confessionis* is different because it is sacramental fails to hold any water. What kind of "sacrament" is it that can operate to deny Christian love, and make it of no effect?

Catholic moralists generally qualify the duty of doctors

[31] Cf. Joseph Fletcher, ed., *Christianity and Property*, Philadelphia, 1947, pp. 193-195. Thus Father F. J. Connell says, "the better theological opinion seems to be that in such circumstances the doctor may (and perhaps must) warn the girl, even though it involves the violation of the professional secret." *Morals in Politics and Professions, op.cit.*, p. 126.

[32] Koch-Preuss, St. Louis, 1925, v. 76.

[33] *Ibid.*, v. 77.

to reveal professional secrets, and some would actually deny that any obligation at all exists in a case such as we have mentioned above. Father Regan allows that in such a case the obligation to protect the girl is a grave one, yet he insists that if the doctor can foresee that some "proportionately serious" harm will come to himself in fulfilling the "grave obligation" he may "excuse himself."[34] Father Slater dealt with an instance of the same kind, and came to the conclusion that the doctor should not reveal the truth, but that he should "counsel" the fiancé to postpone the marriage until cured (or not use the marriage rights until cured), or alternatively tell his bride-to-be the truth.[35] Yet this same writer also discusses the quandary of an English doctor whose patient, a railway signalman, suffers such severe asthmatic attacks that he blacks out altogether. He works alone in a signal box, regulating fast express passenger trains. At any time he may lose consciousness and let a train be wrecked. The doctor would like to warn the company, but his patient threatens to sue him for libel (libel in England being any damaging statement, such as one that would cause a man to lose his job, no matter how true it is). In this case Father Slater concludes that the secret *must* be disclosed, since "the rights of the public must be safeguarded, even at the expense of the individual."[36]

Now, what is the difference between a person's welfare, a single individual's claim upon a physician's charity, as in the case of the imperiled bride-to-be, and the public welfare, as in the case of the imperiled passengers? Perhaps for a utilitarian the difference would be in quantity or numbers, the good of a greater number. But that could hardly weigh as a factor with a Christian moralist whose concern for per-

[34] Robert Regan, "Professional Secrecy in the Light of Moral Principles," *Amer. Eccles. Rev.*, Feb. 1944, 110.147.

[35] Thomas Slater, S.J., "A Syphilitic Patient," *Cases of Conscience*, New York, 1911, 1. 341.

[36] *Ibid.*, "A Puzzled Doctor," 1, 339-340.

sonality is such that "even the least of these" makes an imperious claim upon him. As long as "the innocent third party" principle applies, so that we may not resolve conflicts of interest at the expense of others, a professional seal will be broken to protect a single person as necessarily as to protect a number of persons. Father Slater could defend his discrimination, as between the fiancé and the signalman, only by having recourse to the reservation in Father Regan's opinion. He could maintain that the doctor in the first case would suffer a proportionately serious injury; that the injury to an innocent bride would be no greater than the doctor's loss of practice after an angry swain had denounced him for betraying the private affairs of his patients. In the second case, he would say that the injury to many passengers would far outweigh any loss suffered by a single doctor doing his duty to society, since it is better (as Caiaphas argued) "that one man should die for the people, that the whole nation perish not."[37] But this is only the utilitarian rule, the hedonistic calculus, in another form. Viewed within the context of the Gospel ethic, Father Slater's judgment in both cases is a preferential one, calculating and prudential compared to the disinterested love of neighbor in Jesus' teaching. It falls short even of the American Medical Association's code, a document which is by no means tied to as strenuous a moral standard as the Sermon on the Mount. The Code provides (1940, Chapter Two), "In such a case, the physician should act as he would desire another to act toward one of his own family under like circumstances." This is much closer to the Golden Rule of the highest Stoic morality.

Equivocal judgments like these have their source morally in what Catholics call the Rule of Double Effect, and in what Protestants call the lesser-of-two-evils doctrine.[38] It is

---

[37] John 11:50.

[38] The Rule of Double Effect is, of course, more carefully and fully worked out. A capsule statement of it by Thomas Slater, in *Cases of Conscience, op.cit.,* I, 26-27, is: "It is lawful to perform an action which produces two effects, one

the same device in both schools of thought, whether it is used as a popular defense of the secular state's policies of war and power politics, or by an ecclesiastical historian excusing the behavior of the missionaries who sailed with Pizarro and Cortez. In all such affairs the evil committed (fully foreseen as a tragic or undesired consequence) is condoned by claiming that the good desired is at least proportionate to, if it does not overbalance, the evil. These moralists usually avail themselves of a semantic confusion. A closer examination will show that of the two evils between which they urge us to choose, one is *moral* evil (or sin) and the other is some *physical* or *social* evil (suffering). Now in Christian ethics, at least, one is not forbidden to suffer for the sake of his obedience to the claims of love, for doing good. This ethic certainly offers no advice to *weigh* the ethical satisfaction of acting virtuously against the costs or consequences of doing so, in some hedonistic scales balanced on self-regard and self-protection. On the contrary, the New Testament does indeed forbid us to commit sin (moral evil), and yet gives us no hope or expectation of avoiding unpleasant coincidences or consequences. The Christian ethic foresees that suffering (physical or mental evil) is apt to be a consequence of virtue; it assumes that loyalty to ethical principle costs us something.

Do People Want the Truth?

By way of summary, we may say that in general we can validly assert our right as patients to know the medical facts about ourselves. Several reasons have been given for it, but perhaps the four fundamental ones are: first, that as persons our human, moral quality is taken away from us if we are denied whatever knowledge is available; second, that the

---

good, the other bad, *provided* (1) the action in itself is good, or at least ethically indifferent; (2) the agent intends only the good effect, not the bad; (3) the good effect follows as immediately as (not by means of) the evil; (4) there is a sufficient weighty reason for permitting the evil effect."

doctor is *entrusted* by us with what he learns, but the facts are ours, not his, and to deny them to us is to steal from us what is our own, not his; third, that the highest conception of the physician-patient relationship is a personalistic one, in the light of which we see that the fullest possibilities of medical treatment and cure in themselves depend upon mutual respect and confidence, as well as upon technical skill; and, fourth, that to deny a patient knowledge of the facts as to life and death is to assume responsibilities which cannot be carried out by anyone but the patient, with his own knowledge of his own affairs. On the negative side, we have reasoned that the common excuse given for deceiving the patient—"after all the doctors are fallible and make mistakes"—is not a valid excuse. In the first place, physicians are in conscience bound to indicate that they find pathological conditions and advise treatment only to the best of their knowledge and judgment, not with absolute certainty. In the second place, while the admission of human fallibility always qualifies any claims a doctor might make as to accuracy, *it does not qualify and cannot disqualify the obligation to be honest.* And, finally, we have rejected any distinction between lies (positive injuries to the truth) and concealment (merely negative failure to convey what is foreseen as prognosis and discovered by diagnosis). When moralists such as K. E. Kirk offer this distinction, condemning the former and justifying the latter, they have failed completely to grasp the foundation principles of the ethics of communication. We have argued, instead, that commission of untruth and suppression of truth are alike deprivations of a patient's right; and therefore theft, therefore unjust, therefore immoral.

The only remaining question is: what if the patient does not ask for the truth? This problem may arise either because he does not *want* the truth (perhaps out of fear, being threatened by what he suspects, or for some other reason), or because he does not realize that there is a truth not known to him but now discovered by the doctor. This problem, surely, cannot be regarded as a very difficult one in conscience. In the first case, when the patient has no desire to know the truth and the doctor has good reason to believe that the patient does not want to know it, the doctor should respect his wishes, even though it might well be a proper part of his role to help his patient to want the truth and to become able to accept it. It is no part of a doctor's duty to impose his diagnosis upon a patient or flout his wishes, unless, of course, he has reason to believe that he could not continue to treat the patient properly, according to the demands of the best medical care, without telling him. In such a case, surely, he should explain why he needs to tell (or at least that he feels obliged to tell), and if the patient still refuses to hear, then ask leave to withdraw from the case, urging that another physician be called in his place. In the second case, when the patient is too ignorant to ask for the information acquired by the doctor, it is clearly the doctor's moral obligation to supply it, together with an explanation of its meaning and importance. A person cannot refuse to return his neighbor's watch if he finds it, or at least to tell him where it is lying in the garden, merely because his neighbor does not know that he has lost it and has not asked the doctor if he found it or knows where it is.

Throughout this discussion of medical truth-telling our frame of reference has been physical rather than psychological diagnosis. A great many people naturally raise the question whether the reasoning here would be or could be applied equally to psychotherapy. In all probability it would not, and could not be without upsetting well-tested principles of therapy. In the first place, genuinely psychotic patients fall into Jeremy Taylor's category of "children and idiots," as far as competence to seek or to receive the truth is concerned. If it is judged to be in their best interests, surely the truth about them ("their" truth) can be withheld in the same way that a minor's or dependent's property can be withheld and rationed by a parent or guardian. Yet, even in the case of people who are far from psychotic, suffering some much less pathological disorder such as emotional or personality problems, there is a further consideration that makes a great difference between the right to know the truth in their case, and a patient's who has come, for example, for advice in internal medicine. In the latter case the doctor discovers a truth which is factually perceived.[39] But in the case of psychiatric medicine and clinical psychology, apart from a physical analysis which may be related to it, the diagnosis is one of *evaluative judgment* about the patient's behavior and sentiments. However sound and wise the professional expert's diagnosis of behavior and motives and drives may be, it is, as far as honesty is at stake, in the area of *opinion*. Here, surely, the expert's obligation to tell the patient or client what is in or on his mind (i.e., the doctor's) is not as certain or compelling. He has formed an estimate of the patient and his problems; he has not learned a truth about him. The "truth" of his estimate still remains to be established, and probably cannot be established by any means other than exploratory and tentative therapy. Until it is established it is not a truth owed to the patient, as knowledge of glandular imbalance or low blood-pressure would be. Speaking of the psychological forms of illness and diagnosis, we may say with Carl R. Rogers, "In a very meaningful and accurate sense, therapy *is* diagnosis, and this diagnosis is a process which goes on in the experience of the client, rather than in the intellect of the clinician."[40]

Neither the spirit of rigorism nor of laxism has dominated

[39] This is asserted without ignoring what is involved in the general proposition that truth is a combination of fact *plus* interpretation.

[40] *Client-Centered Therapy*, Boston, 1951, p. 223.

our discussion. It seems difficult, in the extreme, to imagine how a conference of medical men could take serious exception to it. If a seminar of physicians were to discuss, just for example, Immanuel Kant's ethical tract *On a supposed right to tell lies from benevolent motives*, and apply its reasoning to morals and medical care, we could fairly confidently expect them to come to much the same conclusion as we have.[41] We have looked into a subject too much avoided, using applications and reasons of our own, but the conclusion reached is by no means a new one, any more than the problem itself is new.

[41] They might not accept Kant's categorical imperatives, but as far as the point of truth is concerned they could transpose them all into hypothetical propositions without altering the course of the reasoning.

CHAPTER THREE

CONTRACEPTION: OUR RIGHT
TO CONTROL PARENTHOOD

Emancipation

IN trying to arrive at a moral judgment or ethical evaluation, we can isolate four factors to be taken into account in every human act, in every problem of human conduct. These are, first, the motive; second, the intention; third, the means or method; and, fourth, the result or consequences. To illustrate from a field other than medicine, we might look at a politician. His motive could be either personal power or public service, or a mixture. His intention or object—the end sought—would be a public office; this in itself is entirely worthy. The means or methods employed—i.e., the tactics and procedures of the election campaign—might be honest or dishonest, legal or illegal, just or unjust. The consequences of his campaign and election could add up to a more or less wholesome political life for the community. Whether we take motive and intention together or separately, they are the subjective or internal or psychological factors in our deeds; they are *what we want*. The means or methods employed to get what we want, and the actual results or consequences of our acts, are the objective or external or behavioral factors; they are *what we do*. All these factors, obviously, are related in a mutual cause-and-effect syndrome.

It is sometimes said, rather superficially, that the moralist is concerned only with the subjective side of human behavior, that the means are a problem for social scientists, and the ends or results are a problem for statesmen and officers of the law.[1] The fact is, of course, that even lawyers

[1] S. D. Schmalhausen, *Humanizing Education*, New York, 1926, p. 97.

take intention into account when they judge our deeds, and the social scientists are enormously interested in what they call the "value systems" of motives and goals which lie behind social mores and patterns of living. The moralist, in his turn, regards the means employed and the end-results of conduct as subject to moral judgment fully as much as the motives and intentions behind them. The ethical controversy raised by birth control is another matter of high policy in medicine and morals, like truth-telling, and it clearly involves all four of the determining factors of right and wrong.

We have been proceeding up to now on the view that moral freedom and fatal helplessness are the opposite extremes in the scale of human or personal being; that "just as helplessness is the bed soil of fatalism, so control is the basis of freedom and responsibility, of moral action, of truly *human* behavior."[2] Control by men over their circumstances of action is, along with knowledge of their circumstances, an indispensable part of personal integrity. Knowledge and control are what make the difference between puppets and people. To quote Tillich again, "Personality is that being which has the power of self-determination, or which is free; for to be free means to have power over one's self, not to be bound to one's given nature."[3]

This may be the point, however, at which to make one more thing clear in the ethics of medical care. It is not our thesis that in order to be moral a man must be *independent* of nature. He is, on any realistic and humble view, still a creature of nature, however highly developed his spiritual faculties may become as compared to the rest of the animals. He may be *of* the order of grace (as theologians say) but he is also *in* the order of nature. Human control does not imply human autonomy. Our humility is provided for *de*

---

[2] See ch. 1.
[3] *The Protestant Era*, ed. by J. L. Adams, Chicago, 1948, p. 115.

rerum natura because, for all our ingenuity and growth, we are still creatures of the natural order. As Friedrich Engels explained it so wisely: "Hegel was the first to state correctly the relation between freedom and necessity. To him, freedom is the appreciation of necessity. 'Necessity. is *blind* only *in so far as it is not understood.*' Freedom does not consist in the dream of independence of natural laws, but in the knowledge of these laws, and in the possibility this gives of systematically making them work toward definite ends. . . . Freedom of the will therefore means nothing but the capacity to make decisions in the control *over ourselves* and over external nature which is founded on knowledge of natural necessity. . . . The first men who separated themselves from the animal kingdom were in all essentials as unfree as the animals themselves, but each step forward in civilization was a step towards freedom."[4]

In a very real sense, even though it is only a part of the whole truth, we can say that our growth in wisdom and stature is the story of emancipation from mere convention or customary morality on the one hand, and on the other from physical nature or the statistically average effects of nature when uncontrolled by any human choice. Such is the history of women, certainly, and of their struggle for moral status from ancient times to more recent victories: emancipation from domestic drudgery, personified by Charlotte Gilman; emancipation from sexual parasitism, personified by Olive Schreiner; emancipation from political serfdom, personified by Emmeline Pankhurst; emancipation from marital unfaithfulness, personified by Ellen Key; and, finally, emancipation from helpless fecundity, personified by Margaret Sanger, Marie Stopes, and Mary Ware Dennett. There still remain, for all these struggles and gains, a good many influential persons and groups, saddled with the fear of God and ignorance of man, who persist in perpetuating a doctrine of

---

[4] E. Burns, "Anti-Duhring," *Handbook of Marxism*, New York, 1935, p. 255.

fatal fecundity. The moral problem of our right to control parenthood is still unresolved, or at least the right itself has not been won in actual fact for far too many women.

Our march to moral stature in parenthood, to the extent that it relies upon *knowledge*, is of more recent success than we might suppose. It was not until the seventeenth century that Leeuwenhoek invented the microscope. Working with Ham he discovered spermatozoa, and then De Graaf traced the details of the ovaries. It was yet another century (1784) before the priest-scientist Spallanzani traced the movements of sperm, and still another before Hertwig observed the actual penetration of an ovum by the sperm. From ancient times to 1875 we were scientifically ignorant of the elementary basic facts of reproduction.

While the biology of sex was still a matter of speculation and of so-called practical wisdom, many ways of controlling reproduction were tried. They varied with the type of culture and the knowledge available. The list of devices is a long one, but the commonest ones were infanticide, abortion, celibacy, postponement of marriage, abstinence from intercourse, *coitus interruptus* and *reservatus*, castration, and various surgical operations. Magical contraceptives are reported among many primitive peoples, and occasionally even chemical methods or, as among some Africans, the use of tampons. Some evidence exists of practical measures used among the ancient Jews, the Greeks, Romans, Arabs, and Germanic tribes. An Arabic manual of the sixteenth century described some chemical methods, and Theilhaber says the Saracen physicians knew of protective pessaries and chemical suppositories.[5] Fine linen and lamb's gut sheaths were described by Gabriello Fallopius, an Italian anatomist, in 1564. However, such practical yet unscientific knowledge spread slowly in Europe until the early part of the nineteenth

[5] F. H. Hankins, "Birth Control," *Encyc. Soc. Sci.*, citing *Das sterile Berlin*, Berlin, 1913, chs. 1-3.

century, when it gained high momentum. Then, in 1842, Bishop Bouvier of Le Man in France "represented to the papal authorities that the prevention of conception was becoming very common and that its classification among the deadly sins was creating confessional difficulties. The Curia Sacra Poenitentiaria replied that the confessor need not inquire into individual practice unless his opinion was asked."[6] That measure of ecclesiastical benevolence and ethical latitude is by now, by all reports, a thing of the past. Among Protestant Christians the issue was never raised in formal fashion, partly because of the lack of channels for it, and partly because of Protestantism's deplorable habit of permitting moral questions to take their course through the clarifications of merely customary morality and expediency ethics.

Birth Control

It is often said, not at all accurately, that what is called the birth control movement had its start in the population theories of the Reverend Thomas R. Malthus, an Anglican clergyman, who published in 1798 an essay *On Principles of Population as it Affects the Future Improvement of Society*. His thesis, a highly debatable and continuously debated one, was that the birth rate tends to increase faster than the means of subsistence, and must therefore be controlled either by positive checks (starvation, disease, and war) or by preventive checks (reduction, by some means, of the birth rate).[7] He did *not*, it should be noted, recommend the use of contraceptive methods. He only insisted, as a matter of fact, that the population increases in geometric proportion, whereas the fertility of the land increases only in arithmetic proportion. For his own part, Malthus

---

[6] *Op.cit.*, par. 7.

[7] Malthus did not foresee modern mass-extermination warfare. More than ever before, war is now dysgenic. Says a Chinese proverb, "He who rides a tiger can never dismount."

recommended as preventive controls late marriages, or none at all, or continence within the marriage bond. He did not give his approval to contraceptive devices even though they were known to his time; some of them, such as the moist sponge, were being explained and promoted in the "diabolical handbills" distributed in England by Francis Place and others.

The long-run influence of Malthus on our human search for ways to control reproduction was to burden and complicate it, *as a question in personal morality*, with a highly theoretical social policy known as neo-Malthusianism. It is based on the opinion that the world is overpopulating itself, and that we must reduce our reproductive rate for reasons of *social economy*, and only incidentally, if at all, for the sake of personal development and moral stature. As a demographic thesis it has much evidence to support it empirically and, many would say, ethically. Its most general discussion in America of late was aroused by the publication of a small book by Guy Irving Burch and Elmer Pendell, *Human Breeding and Survival*.[8] The weight of opinion seems to favor population control, but not always on the ground that overpopulation is inevitable, economically regarded. A good many social biologists and economists tend to reason that overpopulation is due to maldistribution of wealth rather than to a limited productive capacity, or at least that the production optimum is still to be seen and is as yet unreached and unestimated. Some are opposed to contraception as the best means of meeting the problem; Russell Lord, for one, has argued that the answer to overpopulation where it occurs is "in the soil, not in the drug store."[9]

[8] New York, 1947. Other good books on the subject are R. C. Cook, *Human Fertility: The Modern Dilemma*, New York, 1951; Fairfield Osborne, *The Limits of the Earth*, New York, 1953; and Harrison Brown, *The Challenge of Man's Future*, New York, 1954.

[9] Quoted, Cook, *op.cit.*, p. 31. A powerful work supporting Lord's view is Josué de Castro, *The Geography of Hunger*, Boston, 1952.

Now that mankind is quite evidently living in one world to a degree not experienced in the past, we shall have to come to some sort of terms with the fact of gross imbalance between the ratios of wealth and population in many areas. Human beings have the highest reproductive efficiency of all animals. We bring our relatively few progeny to maturity with great success as compared, let us say, with the success of oysters, one female of the latter producing as many as 50,000,000 eggs per year! Human females produce only one egg every twenty-eight days, or about a mere 400 during their thirty years of fertility! (Human males can turn out several *billion* seeds *per day*, oyster-like.) Whereas women in the United States in 1790 produced an average of seven-and-a-half children each, and the population grew very slowly, longevity and survival due to modern medicine and welfare techniques are such that now only two-and-a-half children per woman are enough to balance births and deaths, and, with the present death rates, five children per woman would double the population every generation.[10] It begins to appear that if nature could, of itself, somehow manage to avoid killing the seed (nature provides contraceptionists with some precedent in this regard) men would before long have to fight for standing room. It was this which led Woodrow Wilson to speak of "the swarming of the English," having in mind such histories as Daniel Boone's and his wife Jemima's and their seventy-two grandchildren and four hundred great-grandchildren, *ad infinitum*.[11] Such, at any rate, are the issues posed to social ethics. The problem of eugenics and population control ("we must have birth control if we are to have death control") is of pressing importance, but it lies in the area of social ethics and outside our immediate scope here. For our purposes in this book, we are narrowing our attention to the area of personal

[10] *Ibid.*, p. 33. By "per woman" Cook evidently means per female born, assuming she will live through the normal child-bearing period.
[11] Donald Culross Peattie, *Journey into America*, Boston, 1943, p. 136.

71

morality. For us the question to be explored is whether we have a right to control parenthood, as a personal action and a personal choice.

The first book in the English language dealing with our inquiry was a rather brutal one by Richard Carlile called *Every Woman's Book: or, What is Love?* The next was Robert Dale Owen's *Moral Physiology* in 1830.[12] But by far the most influential tract of the century, and the first one by a medical man, was *The Fruits of Philosophy; or, The Private Companion of Young Married People*, by Dr. Charles Knowlton, a Massachusetts physician. He first published it anonymously in New York in 1822, then over his own name in Boston in 1823, and about a year later in England. He was fined for the book in a court in Taunton and actually jailed in Cambridge, but he went ahead quietly circulating it just the same. In England more than 40,000 copies were sold before it was presented as the basis of a famous trial in 1877.

Charles Bradlaugh and Mrs. Annie Besant had gained a somewhat uncomfortable notoriety by pleading the case for planned parenthood in their *National Reformer*, from 1863 to 1893. After their trial in 1877 (for selling Dr. Knowlton's tract), Bradlaugh was described in Parliament as the "unsavoury member from Northampton." But the effect of the trial, as has been the case with other book-bannings, was to sell another 185,000 copies of *The Fruits of Philosophy*. From then on, the popular acceptance of birth control was only a matter of time, and of man's inherent drive to climb the ladder of self-determination and self-understanding. We need not take space to trace the story up to the present day, through leaders such as Dr. Marie Stopes, Margaret Sanger, and Mrs. Dennett. They were willing to brave prison and infamy, secure in the faith that they had time and right on

---

[12] This gentleman has a lot to answer for—not only birth control but democratic socialism and the Sunday School.

their side. Anthony Comstock and others had made their cause illegal in this country for a while, by getting Congress in 1873 to pass a prohibitory section (211) in the Penal Code, but the battle has now been won legally at the federal level and in all the separate states, except in Massachusetts and Connecticut.[13]

There are in America today more than five hundred birth-control and child-spacing clinics. State public health departments sponsor nearly half of them, and more than fifty are operated in hospitals.[14] The adoption of child-spacing medical advice has become a regular part of the public health program in various states, such as North Carolina and Virginia. In the latter state there are nearly fifty planned parenthood clinics supported by public funds. The Planned Parenthood Federation of America has given splendid and constructive service to man's moral maturity, with the help of its National Medical Advisory Council. The consistently cautious A.M.A. has a section on Obstetrics, Gynecology, and Abdominal Surgery which endorsed birth control by contraception in principle in 1925, and a committee of the full Association has made a beginning report on the more instrumental aspects of the problem. However, only a third of our medical colleges, up to the present, give consistent course training on the subject.

But our central problem does not lie on the historical or technical side. We are dealing with the ethical issue which is still debated as a serious problem of conscience: Have we

[13] The Comstock Law, putting contraceptive literature in the same class with pornographic material, banned from the mail, has never been repealed, but on Nov. 30, 1936 the U.S. Second Circuit Court of Appeals said it was not intended to prohibit "things which might intelligently be employed by conscientious and competent physicians." The Attorney General did not appeal the decision to the Supreme Court, and thus it constitutes the law of the land.

[14] *New York Times*, Oct. 6, 1948. One Clement S. Mihanovitch, Ph.D., in *Whither Birth Control? The Death of a Nation*, a pamphlet of The Queen's Work, St. Louis, 1947, says there are over 800 clinics in the U.S. He gives no source for his figures, which exceed official ones.

a right to control parenthood, and if so, by what means?[15]
Ordinarily law is a reflection of a common standard of values
and morality, and is seldom if ever enforceable if it does
not rest upon that firm foundation. However, the history of
law also indicates that as students of morals we must distinguish between what might be called mandatory and
permissive laws. Mandatory laws, which require obedience,
are obviously of the kind that must postulate a generally
accepted norm or standard of conduct. Permissive laws,
which allow but do not require certain forms of conduct, are
by their nature *not* grounded in a generally accepted standard. It is on this second basis, permissive law, that contraception at present finds its legal footing. There is a heavy
preponderance of opinion in favor of contraception in most
parts of America, but it is not yet a part of our customary
morality. Many people, especially Roman Catholic moralists
and some but not all of their adherents, are by reasoned
conviction, doubt, or influence opposed to the practice. A
survey of opinion by Elmo Roper in 1943, among women
from twenty to thirty-five years of age, found that 84.9 per
cent favored contraceptive advice for married women, 10
per cent opposed it, and 5 per cent were undecided.[16] A
similar survey seven years earlier, in 1936, showed 63 per
cent in favor. The 1943 poll also showed that 69 per cent,
or more than two thirds, of Catholic women favored it. As
we might expect, 70.2 per cent of grammar-school graduates
approved of contraception, compared with 92.6 per cent of
college graduates. In 1940 a survey by the American Institute
of Public Opinion Research found that 77 per cent of men
and women favored family limitation services as a regular

[15] Willard Sperry, in his *Ethical Basis of Medical Care*, New York, 1950, is
hardly correct in saying he could refrain from this subject because it is "a *fait
accompli*, one way or the other, in most minds" (p. 183). There are indeed
two minds on the subject, with many people pulled back and forth between
them.
[16] *Fortune Magazine*, Mar. 1943.

function of public health clinics. A Roper poll reported that
54.9 per cent of Catholic women, or more than half, favored
birth-control guidance in Connecticut, one of the two states
in which it is still illegal.[17] If we were concerned here with
casuistry in medicine, there could be a great deal of insight
gained by investigating the common evasion of legal and
religious prohibitions of contraceptives, by means of the *legal*
purchase and use of prophylactic devices in the two states
(Massachusetts and Connecticut) where contraceptives are
against the law. It is obvious to all, of course, that the prophylactics have a contraceptive effect as well as a sanitary one.[18]

Religion and Repression

In our first chapter we had occasion to notice that the
Roman Catholic literature on the morals of medical care is
both extensive and technically detailed. In no respect is this
more true than on birth control and maternal health. Indeed,
we might go further and say that the Catholic treatment of
the ethics of birth control is the most systematic and complete one offered by serious students of the question. For
this reason, since the first principles we have already discussed (the desirability of knowledge and choice versus
natural determinism) would lead us to the view that contraception is the kind of practice which has a high moral
caliber (and is certainly not immoral of itself), we might
profit by examining the morality of birth control with
Catholic reasoning as our chief frame of reference and
counterpoint.

The Christian Church in the past has been greatly in-
fluenced by the customary morality and attitudes of Western
culture. It has also exerted a return influence upon it. Indeed,
the two forces are almost inextricable. As to which has the

[17] Paul Blanshard in *The Nation*, Nov. 8, 1947.

[18] This evasion is by no means defended by all Catholic moralists. E.g., cf.
Amer. Eccles. Review, Nov. 1946. As we shall see, however, there is plenty of
opportunity to justify it by the Rule of Double Effect.

first influence, we can only take refuge in the trick question about which comes first, the chicken or the egg. In the field of sex ethics, we find that the clearest Christian opinion has worked in attitudes about marriage, rather than in the subject as a whole. There is practically nothing in the teaching of Jesus about the ethics of sex. He said nothing about birth control, large families, sex perversion, masturbation, fornication and premarital sexuality, sterilization, artificial insemination, abortion, and the like. Only one question, the nature and rights of marriage and the related matter of adultery, is a recorded part of his teaching. There is, of course, his reproof of sexual self-righteousness and hypocrisy, as when the woman was taken in adultery and he wrote with his finger in the sand, "He that is without sin among you, let him first cast a stone at her."[19]

Now, if we take into account the four factors of moral importance in human conduct—motives, objects, means, and consequences—we find the gospels deal only with the first factor of motive, the subjective factor, in sex. In one passage in St. Matthew's gospel Jesus is quoted as saying, "Whosoever looketh after a woman lustfully hath committed adultery with her in his heart."[20] Immediately following is the equally subjectivistic saying, "If your right eye cause you to sin, pluck it out and throw it away." Here we find concentration upon attitude, or the motivation of behavior as the decisive moral factor. This emphasis upon the inwardness of merit is characteristic of the Sermon on the Mount, as it was of the contemporary Stoic philosophy. Many modern psychiatrists warn us against the idea that people should feel just as guilty about bad thoughts as about bad deeds, claiming upon grounds of clinical observation that these guilty feelings are pernicious and emotionally destructive. In this

[19] John 8:7. This episode and saying is found only in the Fourth Gospel and is omitted from many of the ancient texts.
[20] Matt. 5:28.

vein, Dr. Maurice Levine says that this unhealthy habit is based "on the outmoded idea that people can be kept from bad actions by avoiding bad thoughts," and he warns us that "the guilt over bad thoughts leads to a very disturbing and totally unnecessary nervousness."[21] Psychologically regarded, it seems to be clear enough that we do not have nearly as much control over our thoughts as over our actions, and therefore the moral culpability of wrong thoughts is certainly not as great as culpability for wrong deeds. But does the involuntary nature of much of our thinking remove it altogether from the forum of conscience? The two things, thought and action, are related to each other as cause and effect, mutually, and therefore are each parts of conduct and properly subject to moral judgment. Psychological understanding of the ways in which our thoughts are shaped by emotional and unconscious drives—and to that extent outside moral judgment because they are not truly free or voluntary—would cause us at the most only to *correct* Jesus' subjectivism in the direction of a balancing emphasis upon means and consequences in conduct. Indeed, Jesus' own principle of ethical pragmatism, "Ye shall know them by their fruits," is itself a correction. Depth psychology most certainly does not remove motive entirely from the forum of conscience, even though its insights and those of cultural anthropology no longer permit us to say, as in Proverbs 23:7, that as a man "thinketh in his heart, so is he." Nevertheless, this saying expresses a truth which continues to be of real ethical importance.

The history of Christian influence in sex ethics, for the most part, has been one of repression and rigid regulation, at least in the theory as set forth from pulpits and in the manuals of moral and ascetical theology. If any great figure in the tradition is to be pointed at as the whipping boy, a likely candidate would be and has been St. Paul. Like Jesus,

[21] Annual Dinner Address, Isaac M. Wise Temple, Cincin ti, Ohio, Jan. 1945.

St. Paul never dealt with sex ethics apart from the question of marriage, and occasional denunciations of orgiastic practices within and without the congregations he formed in Greece. What he had to say on the subject is mainly to be found in the seventh chapter of his First Letter to the Corinthians. For our purposes we might summarize his assertions under three heads: (1) that it is "better to marry than to be aflame with passion" (vs. 9), but the ideal is "for a person to remain as he is," i.e., unmarried (vs. 26); (2) that sexual access to a marriage partner is a "conjugal right" (vs. 3); and (3) that abstinence from sexuality in marriage is proper only when it is done by mutual consent, and even then it may be only "for a time," not permanently (vs. 5). St. Paul, in effect, advised race suicide through the practice of celibacy since he believed that the "time is short" (vs. 29), that history was at an end, the "kingdom" impended, and there would soon be no more marriage or giving in marriage. Christians, including St. Paul, later on changed their minds about this. They forgot their dream that this wicked world was coming to an end, but they never forgot St. Paul's implied glorification of virginity.

This anti-sexual attitude was perpetuated by means of an unhealthy religious dualism drawn between the spirit (which is good) and the flesh (which is evil), and many Christians have never yet freed themselves of it. By the third century the theologian Origen, for example, won a victory over his lower nature by self-castration. Two hundred years ago Pope Benedict expressed his dislike yet acceptance of the mutilation of both monks and choir boys, but virginity is still glorified, as in Cardinal Gibbons' *Faith of Our Fathers*, in which it is suggested that Jesus chose his closest disciples because they were virgin and when he returned to heaven formed a special band of 144,000 "redeemed from the earth" for the same reason, that is, that they had (says Rev. 14:4) "not defiled themselves with women."[22] In point of fact, St. Paul was not as anti-sexual as St. Augustine, and some others later on. St. Augustine, for example, insisted in *De bono conjugali* that the only reason for intercourse in marriage is procreation. He was thus rejecting the satisfaction of biological need which was the only reason St. Paul had given as the justification of marriage itself. We have to remember, of course, that St. Augustine did *not* think the time was short or that the world was coming to an end, and consequently he had no patience with the race suicide so complacently projected by St. Paul. Robert Burton's *Anatomy of Melancholy*, in 1621, was in this sense much more Pauline than Augustinian. It said, of curing the Love-Melancholy, "The last refuge and surest remedy, to be put in practice in the utmost place, when no other means will take effect, is to let them get together. . . . Aesculapius himself to this malady cannot invent a better remedy."[23] In this same sense, Protestantism has been more Augustinian than Pauline, tending in a puritanical way to insist that sex as a libidinal satisfaction is less than Christian morally. Nonetheless, Luther's revolt against counsels of perfection and his demand that all proper ways of living, including parenthood, could be a Christian vocation stood in considerable contrast to the celibacy-virginity standards of medieval religion. The Council of Trent reaffirmed them by anathematizing those who would say that virginity was not a higher state than marriage.

Leaping over the sequences of a long but revealing history of European sex ethics, we come to the question of controlled parenthood as it takes shape in our own day. It is, for the most part, an ethical issue between Catholic moralists who would control conception by having marriage partners refrain periodically or entirely from intercourse, and

[22] New York, 1905, p. 456. On castration of choir singers, cf. H. Davis, *Moral and Pastoral Theology*, II, 160.
[23] New York, 1862, III, 243.

those who are convinced that the principle of self-control may be applied to parenthood without having to jettison the spontaneity and *uncalculating* responses of love. Even the Moslem moralists, who seldom take second place when it comes to rigidity of opinion, are to be counted among those who favor freedom and control. The Grand Mufti of Egypt, the Pope of the Moslems, issued a *fatwa* or decree in 1937, as from the Holy Office, saying that contraception is lawful when used by mutual consent.[24] This is the opinion accepted in nearly every culture where men have kept pace with the higher moral stature brought into their reach by medical and scientific advances. But we must not suppose that since the opposition to contraception is largely a sectarian matter it is therefore not an important issue in morals, or best left alone. Catholics make up a large proportion of our neighbors in the societies of the Western world, and we are required both by charity and prudence to consider the reasons for their opinions as seriously and thoughtfully as the opinions themselves. A division of ethical reasoning in church or community is not to be lightly regarded, for democracies depend upon solidarity in the fundamentals of moral ideal. If there is a conflict of opinion at deep and vital levels, such as this is, then it behooves us to examine and re-examine it if we are to know how strong or weak are the foundations of our house. To put it aside on some debonair basis such as that "one man's meat is another man's poison," is to concede one of two things: either that ethical convictions are merely a matter of cultural relativism, developing in watertight and self-sufficient contexts; or that, for some other reason, there can be no meeting of Catholic and non-Catholic consciences.

The Real Issue

In order to see the problem carefully we should understand at the outset that birth control as such is not in ques-

24 Jan. 25, 1937, Series 81, No. 43.

tion. Apart from post-natal controls (such as infanticide and Malthus' so-called preventive checks) there are at least five ways of controlling reproduction *by prevention*. They are: (1) by abstinence from intercourse, or continence; (2) by restricting intercourse to the allegedly safe or infertile period of the feminine cycle, a method known as rhythm; (3) by the use of various mechanical and chemical means, a method called contraception; (4) by abortion; and (5) by sterilization, i.e., by removing or obstructing the physiological apparatus. Sterilization is a matter with which we shall deal in some detail in a later chapter. Abortion, or, more strictly, *medical* abortion, will come in for allusive treatment here and there, but it will be seen that its moral validity hangs or falls on the justification of sterilization and contraception.[25] Our attention just now is to be centered upon the first three methods of controlling reproduction. Catholics give their moral support and approval to two of the three methods, abstinence and rhythm; they reject the other, contraception, as morally illicit.

It becomes apparent, as we remember the three essential factors in a moral judgment, that Catholic writers allow the lawfulness of both the motive involved in birth control (to exert human control over reproduction) and the end or object (to exert human control over the frequency and number of births), if there are "grave" reasons for such control. The ethical issue, therefore, is precisely a controversy over the morality of *means.* The intention is the same in every form of birth control, and the end sought is the same, whatever means is employed. It is of the utmost importance to have this point firmly in mind. Much of the popular discussion of birth control is confused because so many people falsely suppose that the Catholic Church denounces birth control as such, which is not true. It has been pointed out

[25] Quite consistently, Roman Catholic law forbids abortion (*Codex Juris Canonici*, 2350.1) along with sterilization and contraception

more than once that the Roman Church "seems to be generally credited with being the only religious body that has 'come out against birth control.' The opposite is nearer the truth. Rome is the only Christian body which officially sanctions 'birth control' among its adherents. The Roman Church not only sanctions it, but officially approves two particular methods."[26]

All Catholics would agree that continence is legitimate. Also there is general acceptance of the rhythm method, based upon an allegedly infertile period in the menstrual cycle and developed by K. Ogino of Japan and Hermann Knaus of Vienna. Manuals explaining it are available with the ecclesiastical *censor librorum*.[27] Catholic theologians now defend rhythm when there are "grave reasons for its use." Perhaps a typical conclusion of present-day Catholic moralists is to be found in a popular manual of moral theology, widely used in seminaries, which says that "it is permissible to limit sexual intercourse to the period when conception does not ordinarily take place."[28] Historians tracing the mutual influence of Christianity and morals cannot help finding some amusement in the fact that Roman writers regard St. Augustine, who became an extreme anti-sexualist after his conversion, as an authority on sex and parenthood, and yet it was St. Augustine who explicitly denounced what modern Catholics call rhythm. Writing *On the morals of the Manichees* (sec. 18, par. 65) he said: "Is it not you (Manichees) who used to counsel us to observe as much as possible the

[26] W. T. Holt, "Responsible Christian Freedom," *The Living Church*, Oct. 10, 1938. The fact that the Pope does not challenge birth control as such may be seen in the encyclical ("Bull") *Casti Connubii*, 1930, in which Pius XI agrees that intercourse is lawful even without any intention of children, provided no mechanical device is employed to prevent conception. He says the "conjugal act" may be followed "although on account of natural reasons either *of time* or of certain defects, new life cannot be brought forth."

[27] Leo T. Latz, *The Rhythm of Sterility and Fertility in Women*, Chicago, 1944. Also, O. Griese, *The Morality of Periodic Continence*, Washington, 1942, discusses its morality.

[28] Koch-Preuss, *op.cit.*, v, 475.

time when a woman, after her purification (*genitalium viscerum purgationem*) is most likely to conceive, and to abstain from cohabitation at that time, lest the soul should be entangled in flesh?" St. Augustine then goes on to argue that there is no proper reason for cohabitation except reproduction. Here we have a clear-cut condemnation of rhythm by one of the four great Doctors of the Latin Church. It puts Catholic writers in something of a real quandary, among the informed students of these matters, as long as they continue to abide by the tradition-and-precedent method of authoritative moral judgment. Perhaps this is why a careful examination of their literature has failed to turn up any reference to the matter.

Our problem is to justify ways and means to *prevent* conception. Continence, one of the two methods allowed in Catholic theology, is a way open to all, of course. We can say at once that whatever its virtues may be in the abstract, continence is *not* a vocation for married people. If chastity and childlessness can be held to be a legitimate vocation for normal people, then they are appropriate only to monasteries and nunneries, not to married life, of which the sexual bond and function is an essential feature. The very reason-for-being of marriage is a repudiation of celibacy. Both common sense and psychiatry provide us with strong reasons for minimizing, if not for condemning, abstinence as a method of preventing conception. St. Paul was quite sound in his views. This is a simple truth about man as a creature, and it has its oblique honoring by Catholics, therefore, in their endorsement of rhythm. The real and crucial issue has to do with one method, and with one method only: contraception.

Incidentally, at this point it might be worth while to refer to the position taken by the Anglican bishops at Lambeth in 1930. At that time they timidly conceded the use of contraceptives in a narrowly limited range of cases, but urged the method of abstinence as more clearly lawful. However, this kind of position misses the mark. An act of prevention is one of three things: morally good, morally neutral, or morally evil. If it is evil, it is out of conscience. If it is either neutral or good, then it cannot be wrong in any case where birth control by abstinence would be permissible, unless it could be held to be wrong because of the end in view, or because of some circumstance not a part of the act itself. But since a bad end or circumstance would vitiate the use of abstinence or rhythm as much as it would vitiate the contraceptive method, what is the difference? None. Hence, with all due respect to the lords bishop, we must reasonably reject such compromising and middle-of-the-road positions. We must either agree that contraception is of itself evil, or agree to its moral lawfulness *in all cases where abstinence is permissible.*

In their painstaking analysis, the Catholic theologians are quite clear and consistent. They rest their case against contraception on the nature of the means. They do not—and we do not—of course accept the view that a good end or purpose justifies *any* means that serves. We may feel the utmost sympathy for the Modern Mother Goose, who relates:

> There was an old woman who lived in a shoe;
> She had so many children because she knew not
> what to do.

But still we should insist that *what* she does about it is as important as doing something. No moralist, Catholic or non-Catholic, would claim that we are obliged to reproduce to the full extent possible biologically. As far as the issue at stake is concerned, we may even concede the traditional Catholic claim (which is another matter in itself) that procreation is the primary end to be served by marriage, married love and sexual regulation being proper but only

84

secondary, and still find fault with the conclusion that contraceptives are an immoral means of control.

Whether rhythm or contraception is a legitimate practice is a moral problem insofar as a moral choice may be virtuous or sinful, right or wrong. The moral quality of a choice is determined (a) by the intention involved, or the end sought and (b) by the means chosen. The end sought in both practices is exactly the same, namely, the prevention of conception. Therefore, if either of the practices is prohibited it will have to be because the means is inherently or intrinsically wrong, of itself. It is precisely upon this ground that Catholic moralists condemn contraceptives. How, then, do they show this *given* immorality? This is the decisive issue.

Two of the terms thrown around much too loosely in this controversy are "artificial" and "unnatural." The Catholics themselves do this, let it be said, with what turns out to be a fine disregard for their own real argument. They do it, evidently, in the interest of a popular slogan ("the moral evil of artificial birth control"), at the expense of clarity about their own meaning. For they do not condemn contraceptives because they are artificial devices. Eyeglasses, canes, and what farmers used to call "store teeth" are also artificial, not provided in nature. Yet in the Catholic view these "unnatural" devices are moral means to legitimate ends because they aid or further ends intended in nature, i.e., seeing, walking, and eating. The real objection of the Catholics is that contraceptives are *anti*-natural; that they subvert or prevent an end intended by nature. Their argument runs quite simply, and perhaps foolishly, as simple arguments often do, on the philosophical basis that (1) it is immoral by positive means to prevent an end intended by nature, and (2) since contraceptives are a positive means to prevent an end intended by nature they are therefore immoral, and (3) since rhythm does not by a positive means prevent an end intended by nature it is therefore morally lawful. It is, of course, arguable that nature somehow and in general intends men to reproduce themselves because she has provided them with reproductive organs and biological strivings, and that continence, or even intercourse restricted to the infertile period, are interferences with nature's purpose just as celibacy would be, and that therefore there is *no* righteous or natural method of birth control. Every non-reproductive way of life would fall under the ban, including celibate priesthood, chastity-vowed vocations of monks and nuns, and Protestant sectarians like the Shakers. But we will explore the problem, instead, on the more specific grounds taken by theological opponents of contraception.

The validity of this summary syllogism depends, as is true of so many others, upon the assumption of fact necessary to its premise. The whole Catholic position hangs upon the claim that nature has "intentions" and that we can know them, and, specifically, that the menstrual cycle includes a period in which conception is not "meant" by nature to take place. Father Connell has put the proposition in utterly simple terms by saying, "In determining the *prescriptions* of the natural law on marriage, good and evil are *estimated* on the basis of what ordinarily or normally happens."[29] To this doctrine it is in order to reply by at least four comments: (1) Clinical evidence shows that conception does in fact take place occasionally in the allegedly infertile period, opening up the question: How many times does nature have to do a thing before we can be sure she means it?[30] (2) As moral beings with a spiritual capacity for self-determination we cannot derive binding rules of behavior from the involuntary and merely statistical or average results or incidence of inhuman or sub-human physical nature. (3) If it is claimed

[29] F. J. Connell, "The Intrinsic Evil of Condomistic Relations," *Amer. Eccles. Rev.*, Jan. 1943, 108.38-39. Italics added.

[30] Gerald Heard, *Morals Since 1900*, New York, 1950, p. 97, remarks that no one knows "the extent, variety and flexibility of 'Nature,'" and that nature is "no more and no less than whatever might happen."

that we must determine nature's intentions by statistical averages, it is no more against nature to forestall conception in intercourse than it is to forestall the "natural" process of procreation among donkeys according to their kind and horses according to their kind (in the spirit of Noah's Ark!) by contriving a mule to help a Catholic farmer till the soil. (4) The difficulties of the Roman position become clear once we see that, on their own showing, there is no possible moral objection to the use of contraceptives, during precisely those times when the rhythm method itself is prescribed, for their own case is that nature does not at that time intend conception, and therefore there could be no interference with nature's purposes in the use of contraceptive methods! *Reductio ad absurdum.*

Later on we shall have to say more about this doctrine of nature, but we might at just this point raise the question whether the modern medical use of testosterone (male sex hormones) and estrogens (female sex hormones), not only for sexual rejuvenation but as replacements for other health values, is not also, on the nature-theory, both "against nature" and "artificial." If it is replied that they are an aid to ends intended by nature, then we can object on the ground that nature's intentions are only to be seen in what nature does, in the statistical average of its incidence; and one such average would indicate (by the facts) that nature intends a real decline of fertility and fecundity between the ages of forty and fifty. Therefore the hormones at least alter nature's own procedure. Perhaps agrobiology's promise of dirtless farming is still another example of a scientific plot to interfere with nature, or at least to alter or augment nature's way of doing things. It seems clear that virility from a bottle and tomatoes grown in water were never a part of what nature had "in mind" apart from human intelligence and human ingenuity. It might be replied that agrobiology is only artificial; it does not prevent an end intended by nature, namely, the growth of tomatoes. But the "illicit" practice of hormonic medicine still remains: if we reason that nature intends sexual activity by the production of hormones, we must also reason that nature intends to stop this activity and to lower concomitant forms of vigor in eyesight and the like, by its policy of ceasing to produce hormones.

A Murder Charge

There are only two other Catholic objections to contraceptives, both of them subordinate in importance. One is the claim that contraception is masturbatory or onanistic, a claim based on a very questionable interpretation of the story of Onan in Genesis 38:6-10. It offers proof that contraceptives are unscriptural and therefore unlawful. The usual Catholic explanation is that "the Lord slew" Onan because he spilled his seed upon the ground (*coitus interruptus*). Onan did this when he was required to lie with Tamar, his brother's widow, so that his brother might have issue. But the Catholic moralists (e.g., Pius XI in his encyclical *Casti Connubii*) make no reference to the law of levirate marriage which Onan violated by his action. It is true that the Jesuit writer Henry Davis tries to have his cake and eat it too. He makes the very ambiguous statement that "Onan was punished with death because he was guilty of self-defilement, *and* employed it as a sinful means of evading the levirate law of raising offspring to his deceased brother (Gen. 38:9), for death was not the penalty for refusal to obey the law (Deut. 25:7)."[31] It is true that death was not the law's penalty (it was public ridicule), but nowhere in the semitic codes was seed-spilling made a sin or described as self-defilement.[32] The account in Genesis merely states that "the thing which he did displeased the Lord." Father Davis reads his "natural

---

[31] *Moral and Pastoral Theology*, New York, 1943, II, 207.

[32] Some orthodox Jewish moralists condemned masturbation as a sin, but they did so on other grounds. Cf. L. M. Epstein, *Sex Laws and Customs in Judaism*, New York, 1948, pp. 146-147.

law" ruling against masturbation into the "Lord's" displeasure!

The other argument is coupled with the prohibition of murder. This one is more a popular form of objection ("killing little unborn babies") than a technical one by moralists. While the "unnatural" argument tried to show that contraceptives are intrinsically evil, this one—that they are murderous—tries to show that they are extrinsically evil because contraceptive chemicals may kill a fertilized ovum with the right to live. (Incidentally, if this were possible it could only suggest an objection to what we may call the pharmacopoeia or chemistry of contraception. It would not apply to such devices as the sheath, the diaphragm, the pessary, or other mechanical interventions.) In this vein of reasoning, that it is murderous, contraception is sometimes spoken of as if it were feticide. In popular slogans we often hear of the "shame of murdering little unborn babies." This argument depends largely upon *argumentum ad hominem* for its effect; it is not to be found in the careful work of moral theologians, and gets no formal support from them. Nevertheless, it is an opinion to be reckoned with in the forum of debate. It is posited upon the claim that a life is at stake following a completed act of sexual union. Is that true? When does a life come into being? When sperm and ovum touch, or when the pronuclei unite, or when they form a differentiated cell, or when the embryo reaches a week's development, or a month's, or three months', or full term, or only after birth and respiration? Catholic moralists used to distinguish between the *fetus animatus* and the *fetus inanimatus*, saying that there was no life until quickening, the stirring of life.[33] St. Anselm and St. Augustine took that view, and St. Thomas Aquinas followed them, asserting

---

[33] Koch-Preuss, *op.cit.*, v, 215. "The distinction formerly made . . . is physiologically untenable."

that the rational soul is not "infused" until sometime later.[34] Indeed, he followed Aristotle's schedule, that the infusion occurred about the fortieth day in the case of males and the eightieth day in the case of females![35] St. Gregory of Nyssa, however, had insisted that the soul is infused at the first moment of conception. The theologian St. Alphonsus Liguori in the eighteenth century argued that there is a difference between an animate (or living) and inanimate (or only potential) fetus.[36] He based the distinction upon a subtle exegesis of Exodus 21:22-23 in the Septuagint version (as St. Augustine did), which made a distinction between an unformed and formed embryo (one with some human resemblance), but the distinction is not even hinted at in the Hebrew and Vulgate versions. To make a long story short, Pope Innocent XI condemned the distinction (in his Proposition 34), and nowadays Catholic moralists generally assert that there is a life at stake, with all its rights, from the first second of impregnation. (Again there is some difficulty with St. Augustine, since it was he who provided the classic precedent for distinction between an embryo *informatus* and one *formatus*, describing only the removal of the latter as murder.)[37] In any case, none of this gives any support to the idea that the sterilization for contraception of *semen virile post copulam*, before impregnation, is murder. In Pope Innocent's proposition we have a dogmatic principle which will have to be examined in other connections later

---

[34] *Summa theologica*, 1, q.76, a.3, ad.3: q.118, a.2, ad.2.

[35] *De animalibus*, ix, or *De generatione animalium*. This Aristotelian theory was a middle ground between the Roman law and the Platonic position. The Stoics believed that the soul entered at birth and the Roman jurists therefore held that abortion is not murder. The Platonic tradition was that the soul entered at conception. The present-day Roman Catholic position has become a shift from Aristotle's to Plato's. (Cf. Roland Bainton in *Sex and Religion*, New York, 1953, ed. by Simon Doniger, pp. 24-25.)

[36] *Theologica moralis*, iv, 4.594.

[37] *Questiones in Exodum*, 80. For the modern position and the discipline based upon it, see W. S. Bowdern, S.J., in *The Catholic Nurse and the Dying*, St. Louis, Mo., 1934, p. 8.

on. It is brought into focus here because it is so often thought to be related to the claim that contraceptive pharmacy may be too late to prevent sperm and ovum from meeting, and thus that the user may be committing murder. Sometimes the argument is even carried a step further by suggesting that contraception is the murder of a potential life (*vita in potentia*) if not of a life in actual being (*vita in situ*).

However, the absurdity of either objection becomes apparent if we turn to look at the position taken on questions of rape or involuntary intercourse, by competent moralists of the same persuasion. Father Davis holds that it is justifiable to prevent conception after rape, and that to do so it is lawful to use a medical douche. He reasons that such a device is legitimate because "it cannot be said with certainty how soon conception takes places after congress; it may be hours or days."[38] Nor is this judgment by Father Davis the only one to be found in Catholic writers. Koch-Preuss says: "It goes without saying that the medicinal or artificial sterilization of the *semen virile post copulam* is illicit."[39] Yet in a footnote on the same page the latter writer establishes agreement with Davis on the exception to be made, in cases of rape, by citing Lemkuhl, Aertnys, and others. It would be playing both sides of the street, as far as this particular ethical problem goes, for such writers to avail themselves of the mercy of the theologians' probabilism in order to argue a probable *delay* of fertilization when avoiding pregnancy following rape, if they then turn around to argue a probable *immediacy* of fertilization when condemning contraceptives. To refuse to interrupt or prevent a pregnancy from rape would be an obvious injustice, but to have a firm grasp upon that much is to discredit the idea that contraceptives are murderous.

Something more is to be said on this subject. The whole factual basis upon which rests the idea that contraception

[38] *Op.cit.*, II, 171.   [39] *Moral Theology, op.cit.*, v, 475.

may be murderous is highly dubious.[40] It is one of the curiosities of popular and cracker-barrel debate on morals and medicine—particularly as to the murder objection to contraception—that the argument has been advanced all along without meeting any challenge as to the bare biological facts at the basis of it. When the author put the question directly to a nationally known physician and writer in gynecology, he learned that there is no contraceptive chemical that will destroy a fertilized ovum.[41] Such a substance would, of course, be an abortive agent, an abortifacient. Thus is any scientific basis removed from this extrinsic objection to contraception. The only way left to maintain the objection would be to claim that an aggression against the sperm, on its way to and before it reaches the egg, is murder; that directly ending one of the two factors of conception is murder. Put another way (and coming full circle!) this means it is murder to prevent sperm from reaching ova or, for that matter, ova from reaching sperm. In such a case Onan was guilty of murder, not merely of self-defilement or defying nature. And nature herself, in the menstrual function, allows innumerable lives to be cut off, if not actually to be murdered. This argument also invites its own *reductio ad absurdum*.

Nature, Man, and Parenthood

Our discussion may now be pulled together with four or five separate observations. The first is that the Catholic conception of natural law is a highly questionable one. No scientist, and least of all a medical man, can accept the view that nature "intends" what always or frequently occurs. The cause-and-effect determinism of the last century is no longer supported by the philosophers of science. Even if they did support it, there is serious reason theologically for challeng-

[40] See the lists of popular misconceptions in John Rock and D. C. Loth, *Voluntary Parenthood*, New York, 1949.
[41] This letter is in the author's files.

ing the idea that God as creative intelligence intends that everything in nature should be accepted and regarded as good. The perennial problem of evil, of course, is involved here. We may reaffirm our earlier first principle that the moral stature of men, their truly human status, is measured by their knowledge of their circumstances, including physical nature, and by their ability to control those circumstances toward chosen rather than fatally determined ends. There can be no moral difference between preventing the natural process of conception by contraceptives, and preventing (let us say) the natural process of obesity by using glandular antibodies. To assert the existence of a Natural Law is one thing, but to derive its content from the incidence of physical nature, rather than from the moral insights of men, is to twist the classical Christian idea into a mechanistic strait jacket, and to deny true morality by submitting to fatality, to helpless determinism.

The plain fact is that the Natural Law concept (*lex naturae* or *ius naturale*) which was taken over by the Christians from Aristotle and from the Stoics, and baptized, was simply that by the mind and will of God there is an objective standard of right and wrong in the universe, and that men are possessed with a rational faculty whereby they may perceive it. In more modern terms, it was a doctrine of ethical realism, as against any positivist theories. The law which was "natural" was moral law or standards, not physical law or normal physiological cause-and-effect. When speaking of the laws of physical or material things, the Stoics preferred the terms "fate" and "fateful." "Natural" did not mean what the physical or material order presents to our human observation; it meant ideal or true or what was originally provided as being good in the creation before the Fall or back in the Golden Age. "To the Greek the natural apple was not the wild one from which our cultivated apple has been grown, but rather the golden apple of the Hesperides. The natural

93

object . . . was the perfect object."[42] The same kind of myth-making can be seen in Wordsworth's *Ode on the Intimations of Immortality in Early Childhood*, in which he suggests that each child obtains the privilege of life on this earth only by losing an ante-natal perfection. In short, the classical Stoic and Christian conception of Natural Law had to do with ethical values and norms, perceived in part by human reason and in part through divine revelation. It had nothing to do with physiological processes. It was the natural (true) law; it was not the laws (workings) of nature when it is distinguished from rational men.[43] But the ambiguity in the term was bound to bear its fruit of confusion. It did so finally in the seventeenth century when Hobbes and Locke used it to describe their utilitarian empiricism. They broke away from the Christian meaning of Natural Law and turned it into a phrase meaning *the observable laws of physical nature*. It came to stand for such things as the law of gravitation rather than such things as the law of the gravity of avarice. In ordinary discussion today the phrase "natural law" evokes anything but ethical meaning. The irony is that Catholic moralists have themselves fallen into the trap of cultural change by trying to set up standards of right and wrong in life, health, and death, with what happens in biology and physiology as the true or right thing ethically, regardless of human freedom and aspiration. This is the final vulgarization of a classical principle. It is a form of Ruskin's pathetic fallacy, attributing will, if not feeling, to sub-personal phenomena.

Even so, a close examination of the facts does not support this attempt to determine what physical nature "intends" by observing what happens most commonly in its working and

[42] Roscoe Pound, *Introduction to the Philosophy of the Law*, New Haven, 1922, p. 32.

[43] Recent research which documents this crucially important point may be seen in R. M. Grant's *Miracle and Natural Law in Graeco-Roman and Early Christian Thought*, Amsterdam (Holland), 1953, pp. 19-28.

orderly occurrences. On the contrary, the facts seem to undermine the Roman theologians' claim that natural sex aims at reproduction. It appears that by the principle of statistical preponderance, the opposite belief—that nature does *not* intend conception—is more tenable! In the 28-day menstrual cycle, only about six days are fertile and 22 are infertile. A woman can conceive, generally, from the ages of 14 to 50, or 36 years of 13 cycles each, giving, 2,808 fertile days in the ovulation periods of her life as compared to 10,296 infertile days. Normal sexuality continues until about 66, thus adding 5,840 infertile days to the sexual span, which totals 18,944 days with only 2,808 of them, or 1 out of 7, fertile. If we grant that nature implants the sex drive and "intends" intercourse (a concupiscible appetite), and further that "nature's intentions" are evident more in the rule than in the exception, it would follow that nature's purpose in sex is much more to contrive intercourse than conception. As a method to demonstrate that procreation is the primary end of sexuality, this materialistic-statistical version of natural law defeats itself.

An additional example may be cited to show the unhappy result if Natural Law is supposed to be revealed by what nature does—that is, by what happens. The Kinsey Reports are positivistically inclined to offer, or at least to allow, ethical approval to what people *do* in the way of sexual behavior. The first of these volumes, on the sexual behavior of the human male, suggests as a sex ethic the view that sex is "a normal biologic function, acceptable in whatever form it is manifested."[44] It is frankly admitted that by "English and American standards" this biological view is considered "primitive, materialistic or animalistic." Dr. Kinsey and his associates set this biological view of sex ethics over against what they call

[44] Kinsey, Pomeroy and Martin, *The Sexual Behavior of the Human Male*, Philadelphia, 1948, p. 263. Cf. also, by the same authors *The Sexual Behavior of the Human Female*, Philadelphia, 1953, pp. 17, 168, 260.

the ascetical ethic which accepts sex as a necessary means of procreation, to be enjoyed only if reproduction is the goal. Thus we have the anomaly of two radically different ethical standards, both claiming to be based upon an acceptance of what is natural. Actually, of course, the facts are that nature uses sex for many purposes besides reproduction, just as it often contrives procreation without any sex at all.[45]

In the second place we ought to repeat that moral integrity and personal being are essential to our growth in freedom and knowledge. With the medical technology of contraception, parenthood and birth become matters of moral responsibility, of intelligent choice. We are able to control our fertility. No longer do we have to choose between reproduction and continence. Sex is no longer a helpless submission to biological consequences. Nor is the only alternative a denial of sexual love, either *in toto* or according to lunar calculations in a sophisticated and doubtful rhythm mathematics. When such calculations enter in, the spontaneity of love goes out. Rhythm is a denial of freedom; it offers only an alternation of necessities, not a method of true control.

For these reasons we have to agree with George Bernard Shaw, who said that "the difference between voluntary, rational, controlled activity and any sort of involuntary, irrational and uncontrolled activity is the difference between an amoeba and a man, and if we really believe the more highly evolved creature is the better we may as well act accordingly." The British Committee on Birth Control proceeded on the view that "civilization itself has been the story of man's control over nature, mainly by mechanical means."[46] It was in this spirit, too, that Sigmund Freud wrote, "it would be one of the greatest triumphs of mankind . . . were it possible to raise the responsible act of procreation to the

[45] N. J. Berril, *Sex and the Nature of Things*, New York, 1953.
[46] F. H. Hankins, "Birth Control," *Encyc. of the Social Sciences*.

level of a voluntary and intentional act, and to free it from its entanglement with an indispensable satisfaction of a natural desire."[47]

In the third place, contraception looms large in the ethics of medical care because all three values—health, life, and death—depend so much upon our sexual behavior. We have already pointed out the highest form of response to medical care is the one in which the patient has knowledge and makes personal decisions. The example cited was the diabetic who administers his own shots under the doctor's guidance. The same is true of controlled reproduction. Modern medical care in childbirth is no longer a matter of stork service; it covers a wide range of pre- and post-natal care. Contraceptives, in this field of medicine, give patients a means whereby they may become persons and not merely bodies. Contraception takes the accident out of both parenthood and medical care.

Our fourth observation lies more, perhaps, in the political field. But politics is also a moral concern, and it is bound to have a bearing on medicine and health. As we have seen, only Massachusetts and Connecticut still make our contraceptive medicine illegal. It is not morally sound or healthy in these states to permit the sale of prophylactics, ostensibly for health reasons, when everyone knows perfectly well that they are used as contraceptives. Can we not grasp the fact that the repeated and thus far successful fight to prevent a law allowing contraceptive advice and treatment by qualified physicians is an even more direct attack on freedom than technical arguments in moral theology can be? The theology merely ignores or minimizes freedom in principle, but such political pressure actually denies it to others, to all. Nobody, in our view, could complain if citizens so minded refuse to use contraceptives. That is freedom too. But supporters of this law are imposing their conscience (or

[47] *Collected Papers*, London, 1940, I, 237-239.

discipline, as the case may be) on everyone else. We do not ask a mandatory law, only a permissive one. It is admittedly a part of democracy that the majority vote makes the law. But it is also a part of the best and most enduring democracy that the moral freedom and self-determination of the opposition should not be crushed out, if its exercise does not interfere with the freedom and integrity of the rest.

This issue as between Catholics and non-Catholics is raised in this form by elements at the heart of the counter-Reformation version of natural law. We have seen how its interpretation of "natural" alters the earlier and classical conception, from moral nature and its promptings to physical nature and its operations. But there is the further and politically more difficult fact that the law of nature is held to be universally valid, and therefore applicable righteously to all, whether Christian, heretic, infidel, or pagan. Catholics do not claim the right to enforce the terms of their natural law upon all others at any time or place, but only, since it is "valid for all," to enforce it wherever the Church's rule runs. Thus, as an example in an area somewhat less inclusive than political subdivisions like a state, they go by the order that their medical ethics concern all patients in their own hospitals, "regardless of religion, and they must be observed by all physicians, nurses, and others who work in the hospital."[48]

Finally, we might close by recalling the classical saying *omne animal triste post coitum*, "all animals are sad after intercourse." In a work on humanist ethics, Erich Fromm, the psychoanalyst, quotes this maxim.[49] But it has its place here too, not because of its emotional or dynamic implications, but for its bearing upon medical care and sex ethics. There is too much sadness after much human intercourse,

[48] *Ethical and Religious Directives for Catholic Hospitals*, St. Louis, 1949, p. 3.

[49] *Man for Himself*, New York, 1947, p. 188. Cf. his discussion of sexual scarcity versus productive love.

and yet much of the tragedy of irrational sexuality could be prevented by the exercise of freedom and responsibility. Contraception provides the way; the sadness of involuntary and unintentional procreation need not come *post coitum* if we want to be men instead of animals. It is high time we meditated fully upon the moral implications of a remark by Clarence Senior about the policy of family limitation in Puerto Rico. Pointing out that (outside of Puerto Rico) there are "powerful groups who claim to speak in the name of God," he added, "They argue that God sends children and nothing should be done to interfere with the will of God. It seems to me that this stand must be challenged. Presumably, God gave men both sexual organs and intelligence. The latter should be used at least as often as the former."[50] We could add that intelligence should be used as fully, not only as often, for men are rational creatures. Either the ethic of responsibility is to be embraced, or we must fall back upon the magical determinism revealed by an Episcopalian writer who once wrote that "God knows when the coming of a certain child by a certain conception will be a blessing. . . . God knows what the parents' income will be when the child arrives, and how its coming will affect the mother's health. God knows all this and we don't; and the doctors don't. All this He can order and we can't."[51] To this ethic of irresponsibility we can only say that sex in the lives of men, unlike sex among the instinctual animals, is a means of their rational and spiritual nature. The rational or spiritual use of any physical function lifts its natural or material quality to the moral plane. Using a popular question in our own context, we may well ask, "Are we mice or are we men?"

[50] Quoted R. C. Cook, *op.cit.*, p. 37.
[51] L. W. Snell, "The Way of Faith," *Living Church*, Oct. 10, 1948.

CHAPTER FOUR

ARTIFICIAL INSEMINATION: OUR RIGHT TO OVERCOME CHILDLESSNESS

Children without Union

WE have been maintaining persistently, as the pivot principle of ethics, that man's moral stature, his quality as a moral being, depends first upon his possession of freedom of choice and, second, upon his knowledge of the courses of action open to his choice. In a very real sense it is possible to regard freedom and knowledge as different sides of one prerequisite to ethical living, namely control of self and of circumstances. Hence it is that when we explore the field of morals and medical care we find that the science and technology, as well as the art, of medicine are adding enormously to our moral status in these fundamental respects. Yet moral growth, like physical growth, brings growing pains with every increase in stature.

It has been seen how these principles of freedom and knowledge apply to truth-telling and to diagnosis, and to the role and responsibilities of parenthood and sexual reproduction. But medicine of late has turned up another problem of conscience for us in connection with the ethics of sex and health—the problem of the morality of artificial human insemination. As a problem of means, distinguished from the ends we seek, it catches us as nearly unprepared as the atom bomb did in the matter of mass extermination and warfare. As an unresolved question, artificial insemination is troubling consciences in the churches, in the courthouses, and in the medical societies. Its full dimensions are certainly not as widely understood as are the questions raised by birth control, although they reveal themselves from time to time, here and there. A conservative opinion, but perhaps a widely held one, is expressed rather neatly by a recent Anglican writer in these terms: "To achieve union but not children by means of contraceptives and to achieve children but not union by means of artificial insemination are both equally wrong."[1]

One of the strongest reasons why physicians in birth-control centers prefer them to be called "maternal health clinics" is that they are every bit as much concerned to overcome obstacles to parenthood as they are to make it a matter of planned and rational choice. A common obstacle to or cause of childlessness is sterility. Less common but frequent causes are impotence and physiological obstructions in the genital apparatus of one of the prospective parents, such as malposition of the cervix or a too-small *os*. At present in the United States there are approximately 200,000 men who are sterile or azoospermic.[2] This is a very considerable number of people to be cut off from any hope of fulfilling their part in the human urge to obey the ancient law: "Be fruitful and multiply, and replenish the earth, and subdue it."[3] A marriage of barren love puts a heavy emotional strain upon its partners. Not many people caught in such a frustration can rise to the heights of marital loyalty reached by Elkanah, the father of Samuel, in his comforting words to his barren wife Hannah, "Hannah, why weepest thou? and why eatest thou not? and why is thy heart grieved? am I not better to thee than ten children?"[4] Without undue cynicism we may point out that Elkanah had two wives "and Penninah had children."

Medical care can help us to defy this frustration of parent-

[1] R. C. Mortimer, *The Elements of Moral Theology*, London, 1947, pp. 179-180. He counteracts himself on pp. 97-99, as far as contraceptives are concerned.

[2] J. O. Haman, "Medico-Legal Aspects of Artificial Insemination," *Transactions of the American Society for the Study of Sterility*, 1947.

[3] Gen. 1:28.   [4] I Sam. 1:8.

hood by means of artificial insemination. (There are also other reasons for artificial insemination, such as the desire to avoid transmission of inheritable characteristics, the danger of improperly matched Rh blood factors in the marriage partners, dyspareunia, and the like. We will not attempt to discuss the justification of artificial insemination in such cases, preferring to explore first the question whether the practice is ethically permissible for any reason, even so definitive a reason as sterility.) When the physician offers his patient this solution it might be said, in the language of the 113th Psalm (vs. 8), that "He maketh the barren woman to keep house, and to be a joyful mother of children." Our problem is to determine whether this practice of medicine is morally justified. The Psalm, after all, refers only to God's doing, not to man's. We recognize, of course, that married couples caught in the trap of childlessness have as many as four alternative courses open to them: (1) they may submit to a life of barren love, a so-called natural calamity over which they have no right to exert any control or to adopt any means to overcome it; (2) they may outwit the frustration by resorting to illicit (i.e., extra-marital) conception by adultery; (3) they may achieve a partial compensation through the adoption of someone else's baby; (4) they may turn to medical care for an artificial insemination, from the husband in cases of impotence or some physiological difficulty, and from a "donor," some third party, in cases of incurable sterility in the husband. When the wife is the sterile partner there is no solution yet available, short of divorce for the husband and his remarriage to a fertile partner. It might be worth while to point out here that psychosomatic medicine promises to overcome some feminine sterility when it is due to an unconscious rejection of the feminine role or to an emotional interference with ovarian functions.[5]

As far as morals and medicine are concerned, there would

[5] Karl Menninger, *Love Against Hate, op.cit.,* pp. 96-97.

not be much reason to make a moral analysis of the first three alternatives. There are conceivable many good reasons why couples suffering the handicaps of childlessness might resign themselves to it, although we ought not to regard mere submission to nature (i.e., the happenstances of physiology) as a highly moral reason for doing so. This was made sufficiently clear in connection with the view that contraceptives are immoral because, as it is said, they are "against nature." There are many reasons in social ethics for disapproving adultery as the solution. The third alternative, adoption, is certainly a morally lawful and emotionally successful solution in many cases. But we are not called upon to investigate the relative merits of these alternatives. Our question, quite precisely, is whether artificial insemination, entirely upon its own merits, is morally defensible.[6]

There is one aspect of the whole question which we might recognize as being in the picture, but only to exclude it as outside of our own purview. In the last decade or so there has been a demand for artificial inseminations from some unmarried women, especially from some of the English women who have been abandoned by war and its destruction of males to a life of spinsterhood. They are willing to abide by society's prohibition of adultery, but through Leagues of Bachelor Mothers or the like they demand that medical technology be made available to them in order that they may have the consolations of a child of their own, even without a husband of their own. Dr. Frances Seymour, medical director of Eugenic Alleviation of Sterility, Inc., says she has given "laboratory babies" to many unmarried as well as married women. "It is every woman's heritage to bear children," she thinks. "A.I. provides the unmarried busi-

---

[6] Dr. Sophia Kleegman of New York University, speaking before the first International Congress on Fertility and Sterility, in New York on May 29, 1953, suggested that the word "therapeutic" be used rather than "artificial," to suggest that it is a constructive and corrective treatment, not merely mechanical and arbitrary.

ness woman with a decent and moral method of acquiring the children nature intended her to bear."[7] This is a medical possibility, not only by means of artificial insemination but conceivably even by artificial *fertilization*. The unsettling possibilities of medical power are great indeed, for now it has been shown that in laboratory parthenogenesis fertilization of the ova can even be brought about "without either the mechanical or the chemical assistance of the male; he could, so to speak, just as well not exist!"[8] Laboratory success has been achieved also in the experimental fecundation of an ovum *outside any maternal body*, and developed to a two-cell stage of life, when it was destroyed by the scientists. Father Joseph Donovan holds that it was murder to have brought this controlled material to an end.[9] But we cannot reach into these broader aspects of the problem. We are assuming that our question about artificial insemination lies within the framework of marriage, and even of monogamous marriage. We are concerned only with (1) the rights of the parties to a marriage, (2) the rights of a donor, and of his wife if he is married, and (3) the rights of the child to be born by the means in question.

The history of this medical art is a relatively short one. *The Hebrew Medical Journal* has suggested that artificial insemination is to be found in Leviticus, in the Old Testament, and in the rabbinical materials of the Midrash.[10] Guttmacher of Johns Hopkins found it was a known procedure in horse-breeding among Arab sheiks as early as 1322.[11] There is very little reason to suppose that it was unknown

---

[7] Quoted Charles Neville, "Is It Adultery?" *McLean's Magazine*, Feb. 15, 1949.

[8] Menninger, *op.cit.*, p. 41.

[9] *Homiletical and Pastoral Rev.*, Oct. 1944, 45.1, 59-60.

[10] "Artificial Insemination in the Talmud," 1942, 2.164. A Talmudic writing of the third century A.D. discusses the moral status of a woman accidentally inseminated non-sexually in bath water used previously by a man, but this, of course, is not a matter of deliberation as in medical care.

[11] Bulletin of the New York Academy of Medicine, 1943, 119.573. Cf. also his *Life in the Making*, New York, 1933, p. 202.

in much earlier times, even though there was no scientific grasp of what was involved. In 1780 a Leyden physician, Jan Swammerdam, attempted to fertilize fish eggs artificially and failed. Then in 1784 the priest scientist Abbe Lazario Spallanzani, professor of natural philosophy at Pavia, impregnated an insect first, next an amphibian, and then a dog which bore three puppies. At the same time, about 1785, the celebrated John Hunter, teacher of Edward Jenner (discoverer of vaccination) and of Dr. P. S. Physick of Philadelphia, succeeded in the artificial insemination of a draper's wife in London.[12] This achievement, incidentally, is not even mentioned in Butler's account of Hunter's life in the *Encyclopedia Britannica*. In Hunter's successful experiment the fertilizing fluid was obtained from the husband. At the close of the Civil War Dr. J. Marion Sims reported the first successful procedure in America. Dr. Sims, at the Women's Hospital in New York, described fifty-five inseminations for six different patients, the donation in every case coming from the patient's husband. But there was only one successful pregnancy. It is interesting to remark that Sims concluded his report with the announcement that he had "given up the practice altogether" and did not "intend to return to it again." He left it to others, "who may have the curiosity, leisure, courage and perseverance to experiment further in this direction."[13]

Whatever the reasons for it were—whether a lack of scientific interest or more of Sims's moral prudence—nothing more appears in medical records until the Russian physiologist, E. I. Ivanoff, published a monograph in 1907 on the techniques of artificial insemination in animal husbandry. In that field the practice was developing for two main reasons: one was to allow control of known and selected strains of inheritance,

---

[12] R. Forbes, *Medico-Legal and Criminalogical Rev.*, July-Sep. 1944, 12.3, pp. 139-153.

[13] Guttmacher, *op.cit.*

and the other to permit a multiplication of herds far greater than the normal rate would allow. Following Ivanoff's publication, the matter received renewed attention once more in medicine and human eugenics.[14] Dr. Marie Stopes claims to have popularized the idea of artificial inseminations for human beings as early as 1918, and in America Schorohowa described fifty cases with twenty-two successes. More recently, Cary, Schultze, Seymour, and Koerner have reported series of cases, as have Haman and Guttmacher. Dr. Seymour and Dr. Alfred Koerner claim that by 1941 as many as 9,850 American women had been impregnated at least once by artificial means. Of these, two-thirds had been inseminated from husbands, one-third by third-party donors. The conservatism of these figures might be inferred from the fact that 23,000, or more than three-fourths, of the 30,000 physicians polled for their experience made no reply. If it could be assumed that the silent doctors were practicing at the same rate as those who replied (a debatable assumption), then the total number of American women so treated would be close to 38,000.[15] These figures have been criticized in the *Journal of Obstetrics and Gynecology* as exaggerated, but they indicate, at any rate, the rough dimensions of the practice and ·the importance of the moral issue it poses for medical care.[16]

"It Is All So New"

No special imagination is needed to see that many issues are at stake, some of them medical, some legal, some social and cultural, some religious, some emotional and psychological. All of them are ethical in one degree or another. Very briefly, we can say that the legal status of artificial

[14] R. T. Seashore, M.D., in *Minnesota Medicine*, Sep. 1938, found that since 1902 only twenty-four articles on the subject had appeared, most of them in foreign periodicals. The bulk of the literature has appeared after 1928.

[15] *Journal of the Amer. Med. Assoc.*, 1941, 116.2747.

[16] June 1943.

insemination is still undetermined. In view of what was said earlier about law as a reflection of the mores or customary morality of the community, it is not surprising that a practice as new as this has not yet found its legal footing.[17] What the courts will decide will be decided for them, in large part, by discussions pro and con of the kind we are making in these pages. There will be, and there must be, a great deal of conscientious thinking done first. It is dangerous and defeatist to say, as Dr. Stuart Abel does: "At least any stand would constitute a bit of *terra firma* in a sea of uncertainty."[18] The Roman Catholic Church is dogmatically opposed to artificial insemination, for reasons which we shall examine shortly, and has been officially on record against it from the early date of 1897, on the principle of "Turn back the enemy at the gate; at his first knocking." Spokesmen for the Protestant conscience regard it with suspicion and reservation, when they discuss it at all, which is very rarely indeed. Many sincere Protestants are positively opposed to it. In most cases, however, their opposition rests upon grounds of expedience and the cake of custom rather than upon any idea that the practice is immoral as such. But we must be quite clear that objections to artificial insemination are not solely Roman Catholic nor a sharply drawn matter of sectarian opinion. Thus we can safely say that Catholic opinion was not the only influence, although clearly a strong one, which led the French Academy of Moral and Political Science to disapprove it as a breach of the foundations of marriage.[19] A commission appointed by the Archbishop of Canterbury reported in the summer of 1948 that

[17] For legal discussions, cf. Vaisey and Willinck, in Archbishops' Comm., *Artificial Human Insemination*, London, 1948, pp. 36-42; J. O. Haman, *op.cit.*; speech of Lord Dunedin in Russell *v.* Russell, House of Lords, 1924 A.C. 721; S. B. Schatkin, *New York Law Journal*, 113.148, June 26, 1945; editorial in *Journal of the Amer. Med. Assoc.*, May 6, 1939; E. R. Griffith, *The Childless Marriage*, London, 1946.

[18] *International Abstracts of Surgery*, 1947. 85.521.

[19] *Baltimore Sun*, May 10, 1949.

the practice of insemination from a donor, not from a husband, should be condemned. The Archbishop obliged in a discussion of legitimacy laws in the House of Lords on March 16, 1949. He declared that the practice, when from a donor, was "contrary to Christian principles."[20] Jewish opinion, of course, like Protestant opinion, is not united or coordinated. Popular interest appears not to have passed, as yet, beyond vague references to test-tube babies and infrequent penny-a-line articles in digest magazines and fashion slicks, or in an occasional scare headline in the commercial press. Serious studies are very few indeed, outside of the technical literature of medicine, and most of them are not given in much measure to a primarily ethical analysis.[21]

There have been only four cases to receive judgment in North America. In 1921, in Canada, Judge Orde denied a plea for alimony in a case involving the claim that a child was born of artificial insemination, and went on by way of dictum, not ruling, to say that the criterion of adultery is not sexual intercourse (as the common law holds) but the voluntary surrender by a wife of her reproductive faculties to another person. However, Judge Orde appears to have held that the moral turpitude lay in the fact that the wife had so submitted her faculties to another "without her husband's consent." This made it a somewhat equivocal decision that provides us with no clear opinion that artificial insemination, per se, is adulterous.[22] In a case in Chicago, Judge Feinberg ruled that it is not adultery, or at least that "artificial in-

---

[20] *New York Times*, Mar. 17, 1949. Pope Pius XII, in an allocution before the First International Congress of Catholic Doctors, on Sep. 29, 1949, condemned A.I.D. (insemination from a donor) and A.I.H. (insemination from the husband) following masturbation; as to other procedures of A.I.H., even following marital intercourse, he neither proscribed nor endorsed them. See *New York Times*, Sep. 30, 1949.

[21] E.g., Jean Lacroix, *Force et Faiblesse de la Famille*, Editions de Seuil, Paris, 1949, takes account of moral factors.

[22] Ontario Law Reports, *Orford v. Orford*, 1921, 45.15, or, 58 Dom. Law Reports, 251, 1921.

semination, even without the husband's consent, is not in itself grounds for divorce on a charge of adultery."[23] On the other hand, however, the opinions of these justices have been challenged, in effect, by a widely reported judgment of a Cincinnati court in 1947 which granted a divorce to a soldier who had returned from the war front to find his wife pregnant by insemination from a donor. The divorce was granted on the ground that it has been done without the husband's consent. Here the moral turpitude lay in a breach of marital confidence rather than in a claim of adultery, as in the Canadian case. Legal indecision on the principles involved is obvious enough. In another proceedings in the New York Supreme Court Judge Greenberg ruled (also in 1947) that the husband's parental rights, in and over children born of artificial insemination from a donor, are equal to those acquired by a foster father who has adopted. In his written opinion the Justice refused to find as to "the propriety of procreation by the medium of artificial insemination," declaring that the question "is in the field of sociology, morals or religion."[24] He was saying, in effect, that the law follows the conscience of the community, and the community has no clear opinion upon which the law can rest its judgments.

Our discussion of the morality of artificial insemination ought to begin with a definition of the practice itself because, like contraception, it is essentially a problem of the morality of means rather than end, of methods rather than the result. For our purposes we can say that the procedure is as follows: it consists of depositing semen in the vagina, cervical canal, or uterus by instruments, to bring about a pregnancy unattained or unattainable by ordinary sexual union. It is assumed that this procedure is preceded (a) by an examination of both husband and wife to remove any physical hindrances

[23] Cf. *Human Fertility*, 1946, 11.14 and 72.
[24] New York Digest, *Strnad v. Strnad*, 238 AD 572, 266 NYS 159—Divorce 27(3).

to impregnation, and (b) by a fertility test of both, to determine the motility, number, and viability of the husband's sperm cells, and the success of the wife's ovulation. There is as yet no way to test the fertility or fecundity of the ovum itself. There are two forms of artificial insemination: A.I.H., or homologous insemination, from the husband; and A.I.D., or heterologous insemination, from a donor other than the husband. A.I.H. is used in cases of impotence and physical hindrances. A.I.D. is used when the difficulty is sterility. A.I.H. may be carried out by the physician or by the wife after instruction from the physician. A.I.D. is the form which causes most of the controversy.

Old Rules Block the Way

As far as formal or official religious opinion is concerned, only the Catholic Church has set forward a definite opinion. It condemns the practice of A.I.D. among human beings. "Parochus Rusticus," in *The Homiletical and Pastoral Review* a few years ago, asked if A.I.D. is permitted for animals, since the practice is widespread in modern animal husbandry, and the answer was that it is, but only for animals.[25] As in other ethical problems of medical care, so here we find only sporadic opinions in Protestant circles, of a more or less ecclesiastical kind. A diocesan council of the Diocese of Northern Indiana, in the Episcopal Church, passed a resolution affirming that, in the opinion of those present, A.I.D. is an act contrary to God's will, of an adulterous nature, harmful to the sanctity of family and individual life, by its very nature uncontrollable by human law, likely to produce more harm than good (a curious inference that going against God's will can do some good!), and by its depersonalization of sex a means of reducing womanhood to the status of a mere breeding machine. This is an impressive array of theological opinions, ethical judgments and prudential morality.

[25] July 1945, 45.10, 775.

Most of the Roman moralists, whose opinions this resolution follows, offer no objection in principle to A.I.H. Indeed, they hold that artificial insemination from the husband, when normal union will not achieve conception, is of unquestionable right and moral validity. But there is a condition stipulated. It must be carried out, whether by wife, husband, or physician, as a vaginal insemination with fluid secured from a normal union. With the exception of A. Vermeersch (*De Castitate*), there is no leading moral theologian who does not denounce even A.I.H. when the fluid is obtained from the husband by masturbatory means, a so-called unnatural act.[26] Male fluid has been obtained from husbands by aspiration from the testes by puncture, and this avoids the Catholic prohibition of "solitary pollution," but it is regarded by physicians as the least satisfactory method.[27] As we have seen, Catholic writers absolutely prohibit what they call onanism (see page 88) for any reason. Even in testing husbands for fertility, physicians may not get the fluid by this means. Vermeersch argues that physicians, but not the husband himself, may induce the discharge of the fluid by exercise of the prostate gland, for purposes of either fertility examination or artificial insemination. He allows it as *analis frictio*. He maintains that the gland yields no semen, so that a specialist may massage it in a treatment presumably intended to have no relation whatever to sterility tests. It just happens that nearby are the two seminal vesicles, so close that massage of the gland will in fact result in the discharge of fluid. This result, since it is not intended, is legitimate, especially since, he claims, there is no venereal pleasure involved. It is produced only as a secondary consequence of the prostate treatment. And, we are left to conclude, since the fluid is there

[26] Masturbation was condemned as never permissible by the Holy Office, Aug. 22, 1929: *Acta Apostolicae Sedis*, 21 (1929), p. 490.

[27] Guttmacher, *op.cit.*

by a happy coincidence it might just as well be used for sterility tests or for artificial insemination!

Now, we go thus far into detail here in order to show the technical nicety of the literature in moral theology, and also to reveal, as we see it, the somewhat tortuous and evasive character of the reasoning required. By such a specious system of reasoning Father Vermeersch imagines he has outflanked the prohibition of onanism to provide a way to obtain the semen needed by "an incomplete venereal pleasure, neither desired nor consented to, arising from a legitimate cause."[28] The basis of this argument is in the Rule of Double Effect, mentioned above in connection with truth-telling and professional secrets. It runs like this: (1) we are not allowed to perform an action the direct and only consequence of which is wrong, for we must do good and avoid evil; (2) we are not allowed to perform an action the direct result of which is wrong, even though the consequence, in its turn, is the means to a surpassing good result, for the end does not justify the means; but (3) under certain circumstances we may be allowed to perform an action from which a two-fold result follows, one good and the other evil.[29] This is the essential content of the rule. If the good end or result of the action is desired, and the evil result is not desired, we may act even though we know that the evil will result with the good. It is on this basis that Vermeersch can justify the non-sexual production of the fluid for artificial insemination, and for fertility tests. No such device of reasoning would be

[28] Henry Davis, S.J., *op.cit.*, II, 209-236. For an interesting discussion, cf. Gerald Kelley, S.J., in *Amer. Eccles. Rev.*, Vol. 101, pp. 109-118, "The Morality of Artificial Insemination." He explains that some Catholic authorities agree with Vermeersch, some do not.

[29] Cf. E. F. Burke, *Acute Cases of Moral Medicine*, New York, 1922. For other explications of the rule, cf. O'Malley, *op.cit.*, p. 15; P. A. Finney, *Moral Problems in Medical Practice*, St. Louis, 1922, p. 8. The rule is set out in St. Thomas' *Summa*, i-ii, q.64, a.7. For a Catholic objection and dissent, cf. Walter McDonald, *Principles of Moral Science*, Dublin, 1904, and an answer by T. Slater, *Questions of Moral Theology*, New York, 1915, pp. 306-328.

needed on the foundation of our own principles. We could take the simpler position expressed by Dr. Gilbert Russell, although he was speaking on behalf of A.I.H. only. As a physician and an Anglican priest he said in the commission's report to the Archbishop of Canterbury that a non-sexual production of fluid, for the sake of the procreative end of marriage, loses its character of self-abuse. "I cannot bring myself to believe that it could ever be God's will that a married couple should remain childless because one act of this kind is required to promote conception."[30]

As a matter of fact, the great majority of Catholic writers oppose the judgment of Father Vermeersch. He seems to have made a use of the Rule of Double Effect that goes too far. They maintain that A.I.H. is lawful only from and following a sexual union. Thus Dr. Austin O'Malley says that non-vaginal inseminations are immoral because they do not effect a copula "which is by its nature proper to generation." Since nature seems to inseminate in this way (and so it does, we must admit, for most of the vertebrates except fish, although nature uses non-vaginal inseminations for the largest range of her reproductive habits), then it follows that insemination by any other means "is an act contrary to nature, one from which generation does not follow in a natural manner, *secundum communem speciem actus.*"[31] This is a simple and direct statement of natural law as it has been twisted into an amoral submission to physical cause-and-effect or the average behavior of brute nature. We have already seen how it distorts the classical meaning of what is actually an ethical concept. Another over-simplification, almost grotesque in its possibilities, is Father Klarman's remark in *The Crux of Pastoral Medicine* that "whatever is of the nature of things is always found in them."[32] The

---

[30] *Quarterly Leaflet*, Ch. of Eng. Moral Welfare Council, London, July 1946.
[31] *Op.cit.*, p. 259.
[32] A. Klarman, New York, 1905, p. 109.

Sacred Congregation of the Holy Office in 1929 replied to confessors, who were concerned with the question as it arises in medical care, that direct masturbation is always prohibited, even for the detection and cure of contagious diseases.[33] This prohibition is said to have support in the New Testament as well as in the Old. St. Paul's remark that *"effeminates . . .* shall not inherit the kingdom of heaven" is interpreted as a reference to self-abusers, and is applied to forbid artificial insemination absolutely if it involves that means.[34] Thus when combined with the natural law theory that a copula is required for lawful generation, this reasoning excludes A.I.H. by any means whatever for the impotent, and leaves it permissible only *post coitum* for wives afflicted with physical hindrances.[35] As Father Gerald Kelley says, "this controversy [over the means of A.I.H.] may go on for a long time, and it may be settled in a short time by the Holy See."[36] We can see that it is being gradually settled by restricting A.I.H. to narrower and narrower limits. There already seems to be no case of childlessness that may find relief in artificial insemination if the incapacity lies with the husband; it is lawful only in cases of physical obstruction in the wife. Before this decision of the Holy Office, two moralists, Palmieri and Berardi, had declared that "under such conditions [inability to effect a copula] the seminal ejaculation would really be directed to the fecundation of a lawful spouse. There would be no frustration of nature; and the child conceived would be legitimate." After the directive was issued they withdrew their opinion from all further editions of their books.[37] A few extremists are inclined to agree with Father Joseph Donovan, who says it is even doubtful if the wife has a right to be fecundated by the

[33] *Amer. Eccles. Rev.*, 101.109, 1939.
[34] I Cor. 6:9, in the old King James version.
[35] Even aspiration of an impotent husband's seed would be excluded.
[36] "Moral Aspects of Artificial Insemination," *Linacre Quarterly*, 14.1, Jan. 1947.
[37] *Amer. Eccles. Rev.*, 101.110, 1939.

semen of her husband lawfully obtained.[38] Ignoring the contradiction in an assertion that we could have no right to what is lawful (right), we would nevertheless be mistaken if we decided that such radical doubt is too unreasonable to be seriously regarded. It is only necessary to recall that in a divorce proceedings in an English court in 1948 both the legal and ethical waters were muddied by a finding that an A.I.H. child of legally married parents was illegitimate! In this case, impotence was held to have prevented consummation and the marriage was therefore void, and therefore the child was illegitimate even though its natural father was the husband. By strict legal reasoning it follows from this that A.I.H. in cases of impotence is unlawful, there having been no copula, and any child born thereby is issue without the legal right even to a name. It is an understatement merely to call this "a preposterous state of affairs."[39]

If Father Donovan's doubt were to be upheld by the ecclesiastical authorities, then *no* form of artificial insemination would be lawful for Roman Catholics.[40] For insemination with the fluid of a donor is absolutely prohibited. It is condemned unanimously and unconditionally. Up to the present, at least, no moralists have tried to apply the Rule of Double Effect to A.I.D. Perhaps if gynecologists, let us say, discovered that highly fertile fluid had a therapeutic effect upon fallopian tumors, some daring moral theologian might try to defend its use! On March 27, 1897, the Holy Office (Roman and Universal Inquisition) replied officially

[38] *Homiletical and Pastoral Rev.*, Oct. 1944, 45.1, p. 60. Of artificial fecundations he says that "when they concerned man and wife, some theologians felt they might be lawful if the sperm were obtained from the husband in a lawful way." Presumably, by "lawful way" is meant *post copulam*. But on his own part he says, "it is very dubious whether a wife has any right to conceive from her husband except as an incident of the conjugal act."

[39] *New Statesman and Nation*, Dec. 18, 1948.

[40] Cf. a plea for total prohibition, in Henry Davis, *Artificial Human Fecundation*, New York, 1951, pp. 18-19. Father Davis explains that only a few hold this position.

to the question "Is artificial fecundation of women permissible?" with a laconic *"Non Licere."* At that time there was no thought of making a distinction between A.I.H. and A.I.D. But with the passage of time the distinction has been whittled down to provide relief for childless couples only when the wife suffers physiological disorders. There is none for either impotent or sterile husbands. The moral theologians may yet make a full circle back to the unqualified prohibition of 1897.

Is Marriage a Physical Monopoly?

We may reduce the major objections to A.I.D. to three: one, that it is the "stud breeding" of human beings, just as unnatural as the breeding of test-tube babies in a laboratory by non-human chemicals; two, that it is a sin against the law of nature, since the husband's copula is absent and yet essential to a lawful conception (in short, that A.I.D. is adultery); and, three, that it is an injustice to the offspring because, being adulterous, it makes bastards of the children so conceived. For these reasons it is recommended that rather than employ A.I.D. childless couples, upon competent medical advice that help would be needed to conceive, should instead adopt the children of others. Suppose we examine these arguments briefly.

The objection that A.I.D. is evil because it may lead to scientific inhumanities strikes at the very heart of the thesis in this book. To be sure, A.I.D. lends itself easily to wild imaginings about a super-race and other science fiction phantasies. Some have actually appeared in print.[41] But medical science, we can be quite certain, has as its motive only the protection and fulfillment of human values. It gives us *more* control over health and life and death, and therefore raises men to a loftier moral level. Fear of the use of scientific knowledge is apt to stem from a reactionary outlook. It is,

[41] *Scientific American*, 1934, 150.124.

theologically speaking, a sign of doubt rather than faith, faith in the New Testament being trust rather than beliefs. It asks us to forsake the widely honored rule, *abusus non tollit usum*, i.e., abuse does not bar use. It is quite obvious that many of those who violate this rule in the case of artificial insemination are not willing or prepared to do so in the case of alcoholic beverages, even though it is well known that social drinking is a prime cause or precipitant of excessive use and of alcoholism.

Should men attempt to suppress their reasoning faculty and the emancipating fruits of it because there are risks entailed? To transcend natural restrictions, to seek ends by means devised through choice rather than by physical determinism, is a human and spiritual victory. With many of us it is a matter of reasoned conviction that our march toward freedom and control is an irreversible trend. Man's moral and spiritual need is to exercise his moral faculties, including those of self-control as well as control over external circumstances. His task is not to suppress and deny his intellectual faculties. Even given the most immoral purposes, it is exceedingly doubtful that the practice of A.I.D. will spread among those fortunate ones who can conceive their children in the normal way. What is the gain (the loss is plain enough) in using A.I.D. when love itself can be the way to parenthood? (The question of test-tube babies by laboratory parthenogenesis and artificial fertilization is another subject, too far afield from the question under study here.) At present, in any case, this objection is more like a speculation for pulp magazines than a problem posed by practical medical science. It should weigh no more in the ethical scales than a similar appeal to the danger of abuse in the opposite camp. Some advocates of A.I.D. point threateningly to the unhappy history of prohibition in the United States after the First World War, and warn that if A.I.D. is stopped by those who solve new problems with the cry "there ought to be a law," then A.I.D. will be driven underground with all the abuses of clandestine practice.

The claim that A.I.D. is illicit because it involves an immoral act—namely onanism or self-abuse on the donor's part —takes us back again to the uncritical interpretation of two passages in the Bible, the story in Genesis 38 and the Pauline condemnation of "effeminates" and "abusers of themselves with mankind" in I Corinthians 6:9. As we have seen, the story of Onan and his trick to avoid conceiving a child for the sake of his dead brother's posterity makes it quite clear that Onan was punished for the deception, not for the method he used. All Jewish and non-Catholic exegetes are agreed about this. Again, the word "effeminates" in I Corinthians is clearly not a reference to masturbation. The original Greek word, *arsenokoitai*, means literally what it says: males intercoursing with males. The Revised Standard Version changes it candidly to homosexuals and forsakes the King James' circumlocution. And even if we grant that masturbation is self-abuse when practiced for its own sake, does it not lose that character when it becomes the method or means to a procreative purpose which is otherwise impossible? The whole moral argument against such self-abuse is that it is selfish, uncreative, unproductive, self-regarding. Surely there is no possible moral sense in forbidding artificial insemination on this ground. It could not be God's will or man's that a married couple should be condemned to childlessness for this reason, and held to an uncreative, unproductive love merely or solely because of a physiological or biological accident.

The second and third major objections—that A.I.D. is immoral because it is adultery, and therefore also unjust because it makes the child born illegitimate—hang upon the claim that a third party's donation is a violation of the marriage bond, no matter how anonymously provided. To reason about marriage fidelity in this way entails a conception of the marriage bond which is purely and rigidly legalistic. It involves the necessity of asserting absolutely that all the reproductive powers of the wife are to be restricted solely to all the reproductive powers of the husband, and in no part submitted under any circumstances to any other's. It is interesting in this connection to wonder whether either Catholic or Protestant advocates of this strict-monopoly view of marriage and parenthood see any relevance in the levirate principle in Deuteronomy 25:5-6: "If brethren dwell together, and one of them die, and have no child, the wife of the dead shall not marry without unto a stranger: her husband's brother shall go in unto her, and take her to him to wife, and perform the duty of an husband's brother unto her. And it shall be, that the first-born which she beareth shall succeed in the name of his brother which is dead, that his name be not put out of Israel." In connection with such donations of posterity from outside a marriage contract, we may regard Sarah's advice to her husband Abraham as an obverse case in which it is the wife who cannot do her part, but still as an assertion of the same principle that it is parenthood rather than the siring that counts: "Behold now, the Lord hath restrained me from bearing: I pray thee go in unto my maid; *it may be that I may obtain children by her.*"[42] Here is a family-community conception of the parental relationship. According to the Bible, four of the tribes of Israel got their start this way. When Leah could produce no more sons and Rachel none at all, they sent their polygamous husband Jacob "in unto" their handmaids, Bilhah and Zilpah, thus leading to the births of Dan, Naphtali, Gad, Asher, all half-brothers of Joseph. See Genesis 30:1-13.

Marriage was certainly not an absolutely exclusive monopoly in these cases, with totalitarian claims. It might be objected that after all the donation for posterity's sake was not made until *after* the husband's death. But in terms of

[42] Gen. 16:2.

posterity a truly sterile husband is already "dead" to wife and child, yet wonderfully alive in terms of parental joy and opportunity. Again, it might be objected that the levirate principle was restricted to the donations of a *blood brother*, a sibling; that it was not an indiscriminate affair for neighborly participation in general. But tribalism of this kind is not exactly consistent with either social democracy or Christian principles of non-preferential community. Thus St. Augustine once explained that marriage within prohibited degrees of consanguinity is an evil because, among other things, it fails to extend the blood bonds of mankind and refuses to make of God's one family on earth a relationship of nature as well as of grace. The New Testament made neighborhood a vastly wider matter than mere tribalism and blood kin. "Who is my mother? and who are my brethren? and he stretched forth his hand toward his disciples, and said, Behold, my mother and my brethren! For whosoever shall do the will of my Father who is in heaven, he is my brother, and sister, and mother."[43] Even if this is a brotherhood ethic (not directly a universal one) it is at least a spiritual or moral conception of human solidarity; it does not find its basis in legal or physical bonds. It is always a revealing ethical test to watch how far people who are fond of repeating "we are members one of another" will carry out this principle in reality, and to see how much they mean by membership. To some it may seem that in Jesus' radical ethic the family becomes lost in the community of those who "do the will of my Father who is in heaven," and it is true that St. Paul warned the early Christians (I Corinthians 7) that the family must be maintained, at least until "that day" arrives. Yet the community has a responsibility to the family, and the family to the community; there is a mutual responsibility. In relation to artificial insemination, when the family as the procreative unit of the community needs

[43] Matt. 12:48-50.

help, it could be that the community's responsibility is to provide a donation of seed, just as the family's ordinary responsibility is to donate children to the community. Sarah's view was that the community should not only donate seed in cases of need, but even proxy mothers as in Hagar's case. Surely if this mutual dependence of family and community, in procreation as well as in anything else, is to be denied in practice, the denial can arise only out of expedient reasons and not in principle.

The answer to the monopolistic interpretation of the marriage bond is a fairly straightforward one. Insemination from a donor is not adultery if marriage fidelity is conceived, as our own principles require, to be a personal rather than a merely legal relationship. In the first place, artificial insemination mutually agreed upon by husband and wife does not involve any broken faith between them. In the second place, no personal relationship is entered into with the donor at all. On Christian grounds, in particular, to call A.I.D. "adultery" is to give it a quality different altogether from the one envisaged in the New Testament, where the highly personal nature of the sexual union is the thing confined to marriage partners. The practice of A.I.D., being an impersonal procedure of medical technology, does not violate the New Testament doctrine of *henosis*, the husband and wife being "one" or "one flesh" (Mark 10:8). Indeed, A.I.D. as practiced today by physicians is vastly more impersonal than the levirate law of the Old Testament, where the same end (children for the childless) was arranged by a means (sexual union) which is a highly personal surrender when compared to A.I.D. The claim that A.I.D. is adultery is a legalism, not a personal or moral objection at all. It follows therefore that the illegitimacy of children conceived in this way also depends upon a purely legalistic argument. Once we perceive clearly the legalistic nature of the adultery and bastardy objections to A.I.D., and discard them in favor of the higher moral standard that declares "the law has but a shadow of the good things to come instead of the true form of these realities," they give place to personal conceptions of marriage and parenthood, and A.I.D. assumes a new perspective.[44]

The only thorough non-Roman study of this moral issue, as mentioned above, is the one made for the Archbishop of Canterbury by a commission appointed in December 1945 under the chairmanship of the Bishop of London, Dr. J. C. Wand. Their conclusions, unfortunately, follow the Catholic line for the most part. The report held that A.I.D. is intrinsically a breach of marriage, that it is adulterous and injurious to the child conceived, and therefore "wrong in principle and contrary to Christian standards."[45] The conclusions depart from the Roman position with respect to A.I.H. since they claim that the masturbatory provision of seminal fluid is not an absolute objection in cases where other methods of procuring it are ineffective. This qualification infers that husbands should submit to such destructive techniques as puncture and aspiration, although the report itself is not circumstantial or callous enough to say so. Beyond the intrinsic rejection of A.I.D. as inherently immoral, this group of Anglicans found further that the incidental evils attached to A.I.D. are so grievous that civil laws should be framed to make it a criminal offense.

Thinking it Through

Now in order that we may not oversimplify the problem, we ought to indicate some of the factors, the extrinsic difficulties, which complicate artificial insemination as a question of morality. There are, indeed, an imposing number of objections and doubts based upon the circumstances connected with this practice; in short, questions of expediency. We can put them under three headings: psychological, social,

[44] Heb. 10:1.   [45] *Op.cit.*, p. 54.

and legal. To come to the conclusion that artificial insemination is morally good in itself does not necessarily lead to an obligation to practice it, any more than the validity of marriage imposes an obligation to marry regardless of circumstances, or the desirability of parenthood requires us to reproduce in all cases, or the moral values of life and learning demand that we go on living without regard to the consequences. What follows is a commentary on the difficulties that surround insemination from a donor; it does not consider A.I.H.

Cautions in Psychology

Our present knowledge of the mental and emotional factors in A.I.D., and of its effects upon the persons involved, is still limited. It is said, therefore, that to undertake procreation by this means is too chancy to be entered into lightly and unadvisedly. Although available evidence indicates that the practice is more general in the United States than elsewhere, even here its very intimate character does not permit a comparative analysis of case studies for any very satisfactory generalizations. Families are known to have proceeded quite successfully with as many as four A.I.D. children. One consideration of the highest importance in the present stage of development is the tremendous responsibility assumed by the physician. The usual procedure, after the physician has determined that the physiological or biological obstacles cannot be removed, is to suggest adoption. Serious discussion is carried on with prospective parents, a discussion sometimes including pastoral counselors or others. If it is decided to use A.I.D. and pregnancy follows, the assisting physician often tells the patient to go to another doctor for prenatal care and delivery.

Doctors seek out donors with hair, eyes, physical and personality traits to match the husband's. In New York and Chicago, physicians have bureaus to turn to for donors. In

England there are two publicly established A.I.D. clinics. Ordinarily the doctor has the couple sign papers consenting to the operation, and agreeing to accept the child as their own offspring in the normal way. Most doctors will refuse to cooperate with a wife's idea that the A.I.D. be kept secret from the husband, although this scheme is a common one with wives who want to keep the fact of sterility from their mates, on the ignorance-is-bliss basis. But expediently there is always the risk that the husband will learn the truth; and morally there is the whole question whether deceit is a tolerable basis in human relations generally or in marriage particularly, especially in matters of parenthood. So much of the initiative and control lies with the physician that his responsibility is greater than many would care to assume. This is bound to be true in the present cultural climate, with its tendency to surround marriage and parenthood with secrecy, and with its shame about non-biological parenthood. It is the kind of problem which has to be conquered in any new departure, of course.

It is sometimes objected that a mother may feel that she has committed adultery, whether or not this feeling is justified in the forum of conscience. As we have been seeing, customary morality is often stronger than rational morality, and it must be admitted that this is especially true in children and in primitive personalities, no matter how adult or civilized or sophisticated they may be by ordinary standards. A great many people are not mature either emotionally or culturally. It could happen that a childless woman is persuaded, by herself or by others, that A.I.D. would be the thing to solve her problem, and then find that it was a choice off the top of her mind but against an impregnable superego of prejudice and prohibition. Here, then, is a possibility of sentiment-reversal in the mother which has to be taken into account, although it is not very apt to happen if we may judge it theoretically or even in the light of experience thus far.

The husband is much more likely to make a reversal of attitude. In the first place, husbands are less easily won to the procedure when it becomes known that they cannot generate. So much is this the case that doctors often make it a regular part of their methods to have the husband press the plunger of the syringe, so that they can say "*I* impregnated my wife." Sterility is a heavy threat to the male ego in many personalities. It places him in the subordinate role of a matriarchal society, he might feel. If the husband consents to A.I.D. and later on has a change of heart, it could happen that he would resent the child and perhaps even repudiate it. Such a reversal could mean a public split in the marital bond, a loss of legal status for the child and mother under our present juridical indecision, a loss of inheritance rights and support, revelation of the child's parentage and much pain to the child. These are precisely the kinds of dangers which accompany such deep feelings as surround marriage and parenthood, and a sterile husband's sense of inadequacy could easily precipitate them. Something like the Old Testament's levirate law of marriage is agreed to occasionally by assisting physicians when they are counseling husbands who are reluctant to employ a donor. In these cases, which are rare, the husband asks the doctor to get a donation from the husband's brother, to keep the blood line in the husband's own kinship group. This means that, if done without the wife's knowledge of the source, the husband and the doctor are put in the position of having to keep a secret from the wife, which is a violation of professional and of marital confidence. These are some of the difficulties we have to recognize because a husband's feelings of inadequacy may not be relieved by A.I.D. Most commonly, however, they are. We ought also to recognize that the procedure of adoption might be no better safeguard in this respect. An adoption would not provide the husband with the satisfaction and emotional enrichment of following through with his wife in the welding experience of pregnancy and birth as the preface to parenthood. In any case, here is a psychological factor of very subtle and dynamic importance.

There is the further possibility that both husband and wife might have a change of heart, regretting the artificial insemination. This objection, of course, is no different from the risk in adoption. Indeed, it can happen in the matter of marriage itself. We take it into account not because it is a serious objection to A.I.D. as such, but only because it is a part of the current debate. The insights of marital counseling make it clear that A.I.D. should never be undertaken to save a crumbling marriage. It is sound only for couples who are well and truly married.

What if children conceived by A.I.D. later on discover the truth? May they not be seriously, even traumatically, upset and broken in spirit? Here again we have a difficulty that is exactly parallel to the one that arises in adoptions. Children adopted nowadays are quite commonly selected from among those whose natural mothers cannot establish their paternity or natural father. This negative factor of anonymity is exactly the same in adoption or in A.I.D. And just as many parents find they are well advised to tell their children, at a suitable age, that they are adopted, may we not say that A.I.D. parents, too, would be well advised to tell their children that they are "co-opted"? Here is another respect in which the principle of truth-telling as essential to sound relationship has its bearing, and on the side of pragmatic justification we can say that the wisdom of revelation, whether for adopted or co-opted children, has been fully demonstrated in the case-work experience of children's agencies working in the field of foster care, placement, and adoption. As far as ill effects upon the child are concerned, it would be infinitely easier to interpret the facts without discredit in A.I.D., with its foundation in a mutual desire for the child between the parents, and a mutual consent to bring it into the world for their love and care, than in the case of an adoption with its history of an unwanted child, parental desertion, and namelessness. A related objection to A.I.D. is that it weakens family ties by its secrecy and deception. This has real weight. It is too commonly the practice to keep A.I.D. a secret among the husband, wife, and physician. No doubt there are compelling reasons for this practice—emotionally, not morally—such as embarrassment, reluctance to make explanations to the child and relatives, fear that inheritance of rights or property may be lost, and the like. But the same questions arise in adoption cases. And there is no good reason why deception has to be a part of either. It is not needed to make a success of either the procedure or the parenthood that follows. The policy of revelation in adoption can be fitted to A.I.D., and in the opinion of many physicians and observers must be.

On a basis of psycho-biological theory, it has been claimed that a childless wife's demand for A.I.D. is pathological or morbid, since adoption would be enough to meet the need. But it is not always true that the adoption of another woman's child, no matter how soon after its birth, will give her the emotional fulfillment to be had in the gestation and bearing of her own baby, flesh of her flesh. It may be that a far more difficult psychopathology can appear in adoptions. We should recognize a fact which, for the well informed, tells more heavily against adoption than against A.I.D. What of maternal feelings if, after an adoption, the wife conceives a child of her own? Gynecologists have reported that pregnancy occurs after adoption with striking frequency. This coincidence was observed by primitive people long before there was a Ham or De Graaf, or Freud. Hartland tells us, for example, that for centuries a Chinese woman would carry a doll when she was barren, and sometimes would go further and *"adopt a little girl to produce conception."*[46] Psychoanalysts offer to explain this as a psychosomatic phenomenon in many cases, due to an unconscious rejection of the feminine role of pregnancy, an attitude which is overcome in mothering an adopted child. Others explain it as a psychophysical event; eagerness to have a child in some way affects the hormones and they over-activate the ovaries, so that each month there is a premature maturation of the follicles. In this condition, the ova discharged are not yet ready for fertilization. When the wife's anxiety, due to fear of disappointment or sense of frustration, are reduced by therapy or reassurance or by reconciliation to her childlessness, or by the adoption of a child, there follows a letdown in the pathological acceleration of ovarian function, and a consequent discharge of normal, fertilizable ova. In either of these explanations, emotional factors play a big part. As far as A.I.D. is concerned, there cannot be any question about the wife's ability to conceive, only about the husband's, whereas in adoption it may have been the wife's failure that caused the childlessness. Therefore, the risk of this contretemps represents a possible objection to adoption, but none whatever to A.I.D.

The psychology of donors is also to be considered. Sometimes it is thought that they may become uneasy, wondering if the children they meet in the local community might not be theirs for all they know. This could be true especially in the case of those men whose qualities have singled them out for frequent donations to physicians or bureaus. However, donations can be shipped to great distances, and the practice of local donations could be dropped altogether. During the Second World War, seminal fluid was flown to Britain from husbands in Africa and on European fronts, when they and their wives were separated and chose that method to guard

---

[46] E. S. Hartland, *Primitive Paternity*, London, 1910, II, iii. Italics added.

against the danger that the fortunes of war might bring about the husband's death without issue. It is a fairly easily worked out arrangement in the medical services, over a wide area of cooperation and exchange. Actually, most of the donors in the United States and Canada are medical students and internes, who respond to appeals for donations in a scientific and purely impersonal spirit. This objection is of such an obstructive kind that it is weighty only with obstructionists. It would be only a rare donor who developed such reactions, as ego-phantasies. The children he helped to bring into the world would be "his" only in a most materialistic and naturalistic sense. On much the same ground, we could, if we chose, object to blood transfusions because they might lead some donors to be uneasy in the presence of unknown blood kin. This counter-obstruction carries even heavier weight now that blood plasma and its use is rapidly making us all blood kin. Once more, in dealing with a question like this, we come face to face with the problem of deciding just what kinship is: whether it is a matter of blood or of loyalty and love. If it is argued that a donor invades his wife's rights, the same principles of truth-telling can solve the difficulty. Experience has led many physicians to believe that a donor should be both married and a father, so that his personality and progeny have had some "proof in the pudding." This is quite probably a sound rule. And in such cases it is clearly a requirement of personal integrity, of love and loyalty, that the donor's wife should be consulted by him and agree to the role he plays. Have no fear, it will be found that there are plenty of twentieth century wives. The testimony of physicians shows it.

Cautions in Social Order

Those who counsel us to approach these matters with fear and trembling point also to the fact that a fecund donor who submitted two donations a week could produce four hundred children weekly, or more than 20,000 annually. Hence there is grave danger of widespread incest. Now, when put in this form the argument becomes a statistical shocker unrelated to reality, since it requires us to imagine that out of each donation the seeds would be broken out of their seminal base by some strange medical alchemy, spermatozoon by spermatozoon, and then medically administered almost one by one, with successful impregnations in each case, to masses of waiting patients! Nevertheless, the possibility of incest—that is, of marriage or sex relations within undesired ranges of consanguinity—is plainly increased by A.I.D.[47] Half-brothers and half-sisters, by the common estimate of relationship, could by some law of averages actually marry unaware of what they were doing if A.I.D. is practiced. Its incidence, of course, could be greatly reduced by avoiding all but infrequent donations from any one person, and also by the policy of a wide geographic distribution of the donations. But the possibility would still remain. A.I.D. does not create or innovate the danger, of course, since clandestine children of undisclosed parentage have always been in the marriage markets. But A.I.D. adds to the frequency with which it can happen.

What, then, are the relevant facts about genetics as a science and about incest as a tabu? It takes no expert knowledge of totem and tabu to teach us that there is a deeply ingrained fear of incest in most cultures, especially the more primitive ones. It is almost universally prohibited in the law. Exceptions only make the rule: e.g., Abraham's marriage to his half-sister Sarah (Genesis 20:10-13); Moab and Ammon, born of conceptions by Lot with his daughters in the cave of Zoar (Genesis 19:30-38); etc. Quite apart from differing theories to explain its emotional power (Frazer, Westermarck, Briffault, and others), in-breeding is not known to be biologically harmful except among stocks which are

[47] One clinic in England has restricted each donor to 100 donations.

eugenically too poor to stand an accentuation of their qualities, or characteristic lack of them. Aristocracies and royal
personages have not frowned upon marriage within a close
range of consanguinity, although unions of half-brothers
and half-sisters were never very common due to the opposing sentiments of their humble servitors and subjects.
This is clearly a matter of cultural bias rather than of biological objection, although none the less important for that
reason. But if people seeking A.I.D. choose to be scientific
in their reasoning, and prefer to discount the danger of
incest as a possible consequence, who is to find any ethical
objection?

As another disturbance of social order, it is claimed that
A.I.D. opens the way to unmarried motherhood without
violating the prohibition of adultery. We have already noted
that some women, condemned by war to spinsterhood, have
candidly embraced this policy. Those who accept the view
that A.I.D. is adultery can withdraw from the debate at
this point and just look on. If, contrariwise, we are not content to accept the legalistic and naturalistic assumption behind that doctrine, holding instead that genuine intercourse
is genuinely inter-personal, then there seems to be no good
reason for objecting to A.I.D. for unmarried mothers on
that ground. How personally real is it, and how truly intercourse, if (as has actually happened) a Montreal woman is
inseminated with a donation sent by air mail from New
York by a professional donor? Can a woman in Montreal
commit adultery with a man in New York? The practice
may well be disapproved on other grounds, such as the
alleged inability of women to bring up children without a
male helpmeet. But this is an admitted objection to motherhood in the case of widows and grass-widows too. Yet is
it not true that one parent is better than none? Would we
deny a woman the right to marry and conceive if we knew
she would lose her husband at once? The military machines

would make short shrift of any such idea! Furthermore, this custom-made objection—that A.I.D. makes unmarried motherhood possible—is exactly parallel to the objection that contraceptives open the way to extra-marital sexuality without violating the prohibition against unmarried motherhood. In both cases the answer is *abusus non tollit usum*. If there is any real objection here, it must be to unmarried motherhood itself. Whether it is possible to defend a doctrine that confines parenthood absolutely to marriage (whether polygamous, polyandrous, or group marriage) is a question in social ethics that lies outside our scope. But however that may be settled, A.I.D. for unmarried women is definitely not adultery.

We have already observed that we have little in the way of information to give us a factual basis for sociological conclusions about A.I.D. Since the practice calls for anonymity to surround the donor, that very anonymity makes it extremely difficult if not impossible to compile any complete data. If we want to eliminate conjecture about criteria for the selection of donors, their previous and subsequent history, and the possibilities of control in the social interest, some way will have to be found to get at the facts scientifically without violating the professional secrecy at stake. In all probability this can and will be accomplished someday, by sound statistical codes and controls. The anonymous element is not a complication peculiar to A.I.D. We encounter it in every research study of sexual promiscuity, courtship and marriage, and most of our other behavior patterns having to do with sexuality. And to keep the A.I.D. question in perspective, we should remember that most of these other problems run on a far wider scale.

It is believed by some that A.I.D. weakens or thins out the kinship basis of family life. Now if kinship is going to be regarded as a matter of common blood, this is a complete reversal of the objection based upon the danger of incest. The genes and chromosomes brought into the family by the husband (which could not enter in in any case because of his sterility) are just as alien or extra-familial as those of the donor, unless he, the donor, happens to be a blood-relation. Indeed, if the incest objection has any validity, the probabilities are that conception by A.I.D. will not weaken the family's kinship ties as much as they would have been had the husband been fertile. Under the primitive conception of relationship, all parentage outside the preferred limits of consanguinity is a thinning out of kinship. Such is the contradiction in cultures which prohibit consanguineous marriage while they insist on blood kinship as the prerequisite to inheritance and property rights. The conception derives, ideologically, from a materialistic or physiological view of family solidarity. From the standpoint of ethics, it is a reactionary view.

Without wanting to *make* difficulties, we can also mention the probability that a scheming woman by A.I.D. could trick an illicit lover into accepting the paternity of a child not his own. Actually, most doctors insist that A.I.D. shall be a joint undertaking of husband and wife, so that this kind of trick could succeed only in those cases where a physician is prepared to administer it to spinsters. But apart from that, human nature being what it is, it would seem that scheming females already have a natural means at hand. They could contrive the same result in a far less expensive and complicated way by arranging matters with a male conspirator. Indeed, he would not even have to conspire; his role could be entirely innocent as far as the trick was concerned.

Dr. Seymour and Dr. Koerner have compiled statistics which indicate that A.I.D. tends to enhance the secular trend in which male births are 105 to 100 for females. In their figures the results of A.I.D. are 160 males to 100 females. Guttmacher, Folsome, and others have challenged the accuracy of these figures. But, if we assume them to be correct, the objection could then be made that A.I.D. opens the way to a possibly dangerous artificial control of the natural sex ratio in society. This is a typically anti-eugenic feeling. On any objective view, it would seem that A.I.D. will be only a statistically negligible source of repopulation, unless we were to be taken over by a totalitarian state of power-mad physicians bent upon manipulating us along Platonic lines of government by experts, in the spirit of Huxley's *Brave New World* or George Orwell's *1984*. Under those circumstances the modes of procreation would be a relatively minor concern, anyway, compared to the many human values certain to be destroyed.

Finally, it is claimed that the practice of A.I.D. encourages quackery and a medical exploitation of patients. Like so many other objections, this one relies for its force upon the logical possibility of abuse. The medical profession, which has made the blessings of A.I.D. available to childless couples, can be trusted to control abuses of their gift. It *must* be relied upon to control abuses in any phase of its services to society. Experience throughout the history of civilization provides ample proof that quackery prevails in medicine and morals in direct proportion to our willingness to rely upon nature and that it declines in direct proportion to our willingness to rely upon the medical arts and their control over nature and its vagaries. When it is objected that A.I.D. gives the physician too much power in the selection of donors and too much vital information about the patient, it is surely enough to reply that physicians do not and should not have to accept the responsibility if they do not want to, any more than they have to undertake a dangerous operation. And if they do accept the responsibility, the information they acquire therein is no more vital than the secrets that many other medical services involve. Why should a doctor's range of professional confidences be any more limited than a priest's or a pastor's? Are they less honorable, or more likely to violate their code?

Cautions in Law

One of the gravest risks entailed in A.I.D. is that in America artificially inseminated children may be declared illegitimate.[48] The English courts have already done so, thereby depriving them of the legal status to press their claims for support, inheritance, and the like. In a divorce action heard before the law lords, Russell *v.* Russell, it was decided that a wife who bears an A.I.D. child has no claim or right to demand legal benefits for her child from her husband, for "even with his full approval (she) has committed adultery without its pleasures." As we have seen in the Canadian case (Judge Orde), the disposition of the courts is to hold that legitimacy depends upon natural siring, and even to rule out the husband's consent to A.I.D. as immaterial (*pace* Justice Greenberg). In the present state of the law, adoption proceedings would be necessary to avoid loss of rights. Therefore some physicians advocate concealment of A.I.D. conceptions, and they have even forged birth certificates in order to assign paternity to the husband. Others, with whom the claims of truth and aboveboard relationship weigh fully, recommend that adoption be a regular part of the proceedings following a birth from artificial insemination. However this difficulty is handled, it is not in itself a valid objection to A.I.D. as such, since it cannot present itself unless adoption is rejected for one extrinsic reason or another. Like some other objections, it is made in

[48] Cf. the warning to doctors in *Journal of the Amer. Med. Assoc.* editorially, 1939, 112.1932. At the same time, the acceptance of the practice by public authority may be seen, for example, in a set of regulations governing the selection of donors, adopted in 1947 by the Department of Health of New York City. Bills to make A.I.D. children legitimate have failed of adoption in New York, Virginia, Indiana, Wisconsin, and Minnesota.

the subjunctive and optative moods. It is a purely contingent difficulty.

Doctors have a very real problem in connection with the false registration of A.I.D. births. When the policy of complete secrecy is followed, the registering physician can become involved in perjury, and that is no light matter. Here is a respect in which the law has simply not kept abreast of medical realities, for it generally assumes that paternity is tied to the impregnator or donor of the fertilizing fluid, no matter how impersonally and anonymously it may have been provided. In practice, the laws governing birth certificates are not uniform even on this questionable assumption. For example, in California the Health and Security Code provides that the physician certifies only as to the fact that he was in attendance at the birth, that it actually took place. From the point of view of *evidence*, it is ridiculous that doctors should be expected to certify that so-and-so is the father. The truth is that any doctor's assertion as to paternity could never be anything more than the statement that he was present as accoucheur, unless women were willing to submit, for the sake of competence in establishing paternity, to something like the primitive custom of nuptial witness, and to the loss of all subsequent freedom of movement. In the nature of the case, doctors could never testify that the putative father, the mother's husband, is in fact the father. This being so, it is often asked why a doctor, in cases of secret A.I.D., should be asked to testify that the husband is *not* the father. Ontario has dealt with the problem, although without any reference to A.I.D., by a new Vital Statistics Act which became law in January 1949. Under this law A.I.D. children are given a better break in terms of reactionary attitudes, because all children are required to be registered in the mother's name. The mother is required only to enter her husband's name beside her own, in the registration, and the husband is presumed to be the father without the mother asserting that he is or is not. Thus all children born to married mothers are presumed to be legitimate. Without entering into the whole question of whether there is ethically such a thing as an illegitimate child, we should be clear that the Ontario law makes a step forward in moral growth.

It has been argued that a physician providing A.I.D. treatment thereby makes himself an accomplice in adultery. This is, possibly, a sound position to take, given the assumptions of the present philosophy of law and parenthood. But it is significant, in the light of this, that such a complicity has never been formally charged against a physician. Such action would be carrying a primitive morality just a little too far. The charge has never even been offered as a complaint before the English courts, where the adultery definition of A.I.D. holds sway. In the end, the sounder ethics of the American courts, which have never asserted the adultery definition, will prevail. Coupled with this objection is the contingent one that both parents and physician are guilty of fraud if children, secretly A.I.D., inherit property left intestate. But this need not be a risk at all if the wiser and better policy of revelation is followed; and the day will come when ethical ideas of paternity will be patterned, not on physiological nature, but on moral choice and freedom.

By the strict logic of a primitive doctrine of paternity, and under the laws governing the responsibility of putative fathers in cases of illegitimacy and unmarried mothers, the donor in A.I.D. cases would be liable for the support of the children born of his donations. If a donor has made several donations, and his paternity was established in court, his responsibilities could be a ruinous thing for him financially. The policy of anonymity is so zealously guarded by physicians, however, that the risk is rather academic unless the principle of privileged communication is to be qualified so radically that it becomes of none effect. And as in the case of the physician's own alleged complicity, the courts nowhere have sought to assert or to prove such an indictment of donors. It would be beyond all common sense.

Where the Matter Stands

To draw together the points we have made and the reasoning we have used, suppose we recapitulate briefly. We have made a fair effort to indicate plainly the limitations of this analysis, especially as to the subject's many elements of conjecture. We have focused our attention directly upon the question, as a moral problem, whether the practice of artificial insemination, both on the patient's part and the physician's, is inherently and intrinsically wrong. We have developed the view that it is morally lawful, and we have done this mainly in the form of a counter-argument to the Catholic case, which we found to be based on faulty assumptions. Law, psychology, and social interest, however, should prepare us to hear it claimed that the extrinsic factors are weighty enough to make the practice of A.I.D. inexpedient. This is a question of prudence, however, and not of ethical validity. It seems, on our analysis, that there are no objections to A.I.H.

It is worth repeating that the Catholic moralists, or at least a majority of them, have no objection to A.I.H. But their grounds of defense are such as to provide relief of childlessness only in cases where the difficulty is physiological, not biological. Their insistence upon a copula for lawful generation denies relief in cases of impotence. There is no hope in their ethics for couples frustrated by male sterility. It makes no difference how great or how legitimate the desire for a child. Nor is there any moral value or weight attached to the faithfulness of a man and wife within their bonds of marriage fidelity. The ethical proscription of any self-induced fluid for the purpose is a tragic legalism, exceeded only by the legalism of an attempt (like Vermeersch's) to circumvent it without repudiating it.

As we have seen, much of the force of the view we defend depends upon whether we have started with valid first principles. We have asserted two things, fundamentally: (1) that the fidelity of marriage is a *personal* bond between husband and wife, not primarily a legal contract, and (2) that parenthood is a *moral* relationship with children, not a material or merely physical relationship. The claim that A.I.D. is immoral rests upon the view that marriage is an absolute generative, as well as sexual, monopoly; and that parenthood is an essentially, if not solely, physiological partnership. Neither of these ideas is compatible with a morality that welcomes emancipation from natural necessity, or with the Christian ethic which raises morality to the level of love (a *personal* bond), above the determinism of nature and the rigidities of the law as distinguished from love. There is at least a left-handed reassurance for advocates of A.I.D. in an editorial of the *London Church Times* (Anglican), which said that "clear thinking is required to meet the arguments used in A.I.D.'s favor."[49]

We might make one final point, of a sociological rather than ethical kind. Although the birth rate in the Western democracies has risen of late, many experts believe that this is only a temporary variation in a long-term crude rate of decline. The illegitimate birth rate has turned downward since the end of the Second World War, and it always tends to anticipate or follow the legitimate rate. At the same time, the incidence of sterility seems to be increasing. These two trends are converging lines. If they continue, they must reach a point at which there will be fewer children available for adoption than would-be parents wanting them. For this reason, if not for moral and personal reasons, the pressure for A.I.D. is likely to increase. Normally, all of us want children. Not many married couples will be content with a permanently barren love. The end or purpose of parenthood

[49] Sep. 23, 1949.

is implanted in us biologically and emotionally, to say nothing of the spiritual need for sharing. The question is: what means shall we employ to satisfy it? As Aldous Huxley says in *Ape and Essence*, "Ends are ape chosen; only the means are man's."[50]

[50] New York, 1948, p. 45.

CHAPTER FIVE

STERILIZATION: OUR RIGHT
TO FORECLOSE PARENTHOOD

Birthright of the Unborn

Our courts of law in this enlightened country will not knowingly grant a decree for an insane, feeble-minded, or otherwise unfit person to adopt a child. Their objection in such cases would rest upon moral grounds: a child has a right to a minimum standard of care and security, and parents, whether natural or adoptive, are obliged in conscience to possess the competence necessary to render to their children their dues. On this view of the obligations of parenthood, we cannot avoid asking the question: if the law will not permit unfit persons to adopt a child, why should it permit them to conceive and bring forth a child?

This is no academic inquiry. Courts of common pleas, child-placement agencies, and private practitioners of medicine are faced with the problem every day. It is a practical issue of frequent occurrence in medical care and sex ethics. It is fundamentally a moral question, only secondarily a legal one, for the law seeks only to express and sanction the measured and mature conscience of the community. The assumption or major premise in this chapter will be, therefore, in the words of the White House Conference on Child Health and Protection, in 1930: "There should be no child in America that has not the complete *birthright* of a sound mind in a sound body, and that has not been born under proper conditions." As we shall see, "proper conditions" are not a matter of ethical agreement in America. The phrase suggests matters of economic security, housing, educational opportunities, and other social conditions of life and livelihood. These things are of vital moral importance, assuredly, even though they lie more fully in the field of social ethics than our investigation is intended to go. But sound minds and sound bodies often are as much dependent upon a child's conception and inheritance as upon his tutelage and opportunities. They are obviously and directly at stake in the morals of medical care.

Up to this point in these pages we have been trying to defend the primary moral claim to personal integrity. We have located that integrity in our human freedom of choice and in our knowledge of the facts that bear upon our choices. In connection with contraception and artificial insemination we challenged any attempt to assert the right of nature to overrule human self-determination. We have denied that there is any rigid and unalterable obligation to abide by either physical or human norms and standards regardless of circumstances or rational insight. In this spirit we have repudiated a fallacious idea of the Natural Law which forbids married people to become parents because nature has made a would-be father sterile, or which forbids parents to select the time and conditions of a child's conception and birth. Theologically speaking, it appears that this amounts to denying that there are any divine rights or duties either expressed or revealed in natural or physical necessities, or in any other way than through personal (i.e., human) experience and decision.

Our next task is to see whether the reasoning applied to contraception and artificial insemination will apply with equal force to sterilization. If our procreation is such as to render even the most devoted parenthood a futile and tragic enterprise, have we a right to choose to cease reproducing altogether, to foreclose any possibility of its occurrence? The divine right of kings was once as firmly fixed as any canon of the church, but it has disappeared before the march of enlightenment and democracy's principle of corporate self-determination. The time is coming when the dictum of the divine right of parenthood will likewise give way and be replaced by the *child's* divine right to be born in freedom from disease and defect.

Sterilization as a matter of medical care or surgery is a modern achievement. In all practical terms, sterilization is a twentieth-century development. It had its earliest beginning in pre-medical fashion as either a form of punishment or a device accessory to prostitution (*mulier excisa*). What was in pre-scientific times called unsexing people was, simply, castration: an excision of the glands. There is evidence to show that this practice was followed by all peoples at all times.[1] It was introduced into England by the Normans, as a punitive measure, mainly as a punishment for rape. Negroes in America in the pre-Civil War days of chattel slavery were often treated by their owners in this manner, either as a punishment for disobedience and crime, or in order to develop sturdier field hands by a kind of negative selection. Mohammedans have mutilated boys in order to provide overseers for their harems.[2]

This custom of creating eunuchs was a common one in the Near East prior to the appearance of the Moslem religion and of Christianity. The Old Testament abounds in references to such misused persons.[3] The treasury officer of Queen Candace of the Ethiopians, converted by Philip on the Gaza road to Jerusalem, was a eunuch.[4] The custom was so common, indeed, that Jesus used it as an analogy in his remark that some are born eunuchs, some are compelled to be, and "some have made themselves eunuchs for the kingdom of heaven's sake."[5] Assyrians, Chinese, Hindus, Egyptians, Greeks, Persians, Romans—they all desexed their captives,

[1] J. H. Landman, *Human Sterilization: The History of the Sexual Sterilization Movement*, New York, 1932, pp. 51-53.

[2] Besides Landman, cf. A. F. Guttmacher, *Life in the Making*, New York, 1933, pp. 107-111.

[3] II Kings 9:32; Isa. 56:4; Jer. 38:7; Dan. 1:3; etc.

[4] Acts 8:26-39.   [5] Matt. 19:12.

criminals, and slaves for penal reasons. In Java, the Malay Peninsula, the Philippines, Australasia, the North and South Amerindians, the aborigines almost universally have practiced it for the sake of religion. It has even been a regular cultic practice of the Skoptics, a Christian sect in modern Russia, performed as a religious rite by one faithful believer upon another.

However, sterilization in any rational and responsible form, as a medical art, is a distinctly recent procedure. The old castrative methods are a thing of the past, except as an aberration of primitive personalities hanging on in modern times. They were supplanted medically about the turn of this century with new techniques worked out by medical men for medical reasons. The first was reported by a Swiss surgeon in 1897, called "salpingectomy," a device to sterilize women. It was so called because it consists in cutting the fallopian tubes (salpinx), an operation of no more serious proportions than an appendectomy.[6] The next innovation, developed in America in 1899, was a procedure known as "vasectomy." It is an ideally simple method of severing two ducts called the *vasa deferentia*, an operation that can be performed in ten minutes in a surgeon's office, although most doctors prefer a hospital stay of a day or two. It was worked out by Dr. H. C. Sharp, official physician at the Indiana State Reformatory. He first did it illegally, and continued to do it on that basis until a supporting law was passed in the state legislature in 1907.[7] In these vasectomies nothing is removed from the body; they are relatively uncomplicated operations needing only a local anesthetic. They are, therefore, "altogether different from castration which removes

[6] *Your Questions about Sterilization Answered*, Birthright, Inc., Princeton, N.J., 1944, p. 11. Reliable statistical and general data are available through the Human Betterment Assoc., in New York City.

[7] Cf. his own account, *The Sterilization of Degenerates*, a pamphlet of no date, about 1908.

the ovaries or testicles."[8] It is worth some thought that both of these medical achievements came about in democratic countries. They were not spawned under dictatorships or carried out behind barbed wire. There is also significance in the fact that, at least in America, medical men charged with the care of degenerates and criminal repeaters, and gynecologists in private practice, were not afraid to devise these methods and put them to work even in the absence of enabling legislation. Let it also be said, however, that they did so in the face of customary morality. The first public law proposed was in Michigan, in 1897, but it failed to pass. The first to be enacted was in Indiana, in 1907.

We find sterilization being advocated for three different reasons, or to serve three different purposes, each of which, it is claimed, is a just and good purpose. The first of these is a *therapeutic* one: for example, as a means of removing a diseased member or organ of the genital apparatus, the member to be removed being essential to the generative function. Furthermore, under therapeutic sterilization non-Roman Catholics may also have the motive or purpose of preventing further conception in cases where medical advice gives warning that pregnancy will endanger or certainly destroy the mother's life, even though the organ removed or dysfunctioned is not diseased. The second cause is the *eugenic* one: for example, to prevent the procreation of a child who would be defective or diseased according to the reasonable predictions of genetics and medicine. The third cause is *punitive*: for example, to punish a sex offender or to make it impossible for him to repeat the offense. We shall consider these three reasons in turn—the therapeutic, the eugenic, and the punitive—examining the first in some detail and the others more briefly, to see what ethical values are at stake.

[8] C. J. Gamble, M.D., in *Hygeia*, the health magazine of the A.M.A., Jan. 1948.

A Moral Roadblock

In earlier chapters our discussion often took the form of a dialectic discussion with Catholic opinion. This was as much —or more—because moralists in that communion have accumulated the most thoroughgoing literature and serious analysis on the subject as it was because our own principles and opinions stand in some basic respects over against theirs. The Roman Catholic views, incidentally, have sometimes been put forward quite ably by laymen and physicians, without using the systematic language of moral theology.[9] Therefore in discussing sterilization for therapeutic reasons, we can find some happy relief in the fact that the opinions of Catholic moralists are, in this case, at least in partial agreement with the position we have developed. Therapeutic sterilization may be said to be of two kinds, curative and preventive. Now, according to Catholic moral theologians, the curative form (to cure disease) is permissible, or morally licit, but the preventive form (to prevent a diseased baby) they condemn firmly and positively. From our own vantage ground, of course, it will seem very odd indeed that anybody could tolerate curative or corrective medicine and at the same time denounce preventive medicine. Yet here in sterilization we have a case of just that fine distinction. Koch-Preuss says in his standard text, "Vasectomy and the excision of the uterus or ovaries are operations which, though permissible when necessary for the direct preservation of life or health, would be sinful if performed for the sole purpose of superinducing sterility."[10]

The Roman permission of curative sterilizations is granted on the principle, to quote Father Davis, that "the body may not be mutilated unless mutilation is the only available means of saving the rest of the body, i.e., its life or health. . . . But

[9] E.g., Halliday Sutherland, M.D., *Laws of Life*, New York, 1936.
[10] *Op.cit.*, III, 84. So also Sabetti-Barrett, n. 267; Noldin, II, 352; O'Malley, 244 sq.; Davis, II, 163ff.; etc.

since life is better than a member of the body, the latter may be sacrificed, if necessary, to save the whole body."[11] It follows, for example, that if a cancerous prostate gland threatens a man's life, he may rightfully undergo radical therapy on that organ, even though sterilization is a by-product of the treatment. Or again, if sarcoma of an ovary or womb is found to be threatening a woman's life, the organ may be removed. After all, as we have already seen, St. Thomas Aquinas held that "a part may be sacrificed to save the whole." This follows under the Rule of Double Effect as well, for although sterilization is a sin, it is always lawful to preserve a life, and therefore in such operations if the intention is to save life and not to sterilize there is no culpability for sin. But what is the position, it will be asked, if the medical need for a curative sterilization arises in the form of a hysterectomy during a pregnancy, since in this case another life is at stake (at least, according to Innocent XI's Proposition 34)?

In our foregoing discussions we have traced out the theory that a life and soul, with all human rights, both natural and supernatural, is *in being* immediately following fertilization in the mother. Universally, for a thousand years, Christians held firmly to the opinion of Fulgentius in the sixth century, "It is to be believed beyond doubt," he said, ". . . infants, whether they die in their mother's womb, or after they are born, without baptism . . . are punished with an everlasting punishment."[12] This is why there is the following rule in Catholic hospitals: "In the event of an operation for the removal of a diseased organ containing a living fetus, the fetus should be extracted and baptized before the excised organ is sent to the pathologist."[13] The belief is, therefore,

[11] *Op.cit.*, II, 156.

[12] *De fide*, 27. Cited Ed. Westermarck, *Christianity and Morals*, New York, 1939, p. 244.

[13] *Ethical and Religious Directives for Catholic Hospitals*, Catholic Hospital Assoc., St. Louis 4, Mo., p. 3.

that both a mortal life and an immortal soul are in jeopardy if the physician carries out a curative, therapeutic abortion. We can illustrate the morality of this position by looking at the problem as it is presented in one particular case of abortion, known as ectopic pregnancy. We use the case, as almost all ethical analysts do, because of its unique illustrative value. Ectopic pregnancies are a pathological condition in which a fertilized egg is lodged in a fallopian tube and threatens death to both embryo and mother if it is allowed to continue. This situation will make manifest all the intricacies and involutions of medical ethics when it is approached in a dogmatic and legalistic way, and when supported by a naturalistic theory of right and wrong. The problem will also show the fallacies of such an approach, when examined in the light of rational rather than theocratic moral principles.

First, however, it might be of interest to the theologically minded if we briefly outline the traditional Christian ideology of childbirth and its hazards. This summary is based upon Father Klarman's account in his *The Crux of Pastoral Medicine: The Perils of Embryonic Man*. It is fully as traditional, perhaps even contemporary, in Protestantism as in Catholicism. Therapeutic abortions, says Father Klarman, are ideologically impossible to justify because: (1) the source of all human misery is in original sin; (2) in no creature is it more manifest than in woman, who first disobeyed God; (3) the fury of that case was in part abated by the divine charity introduced by Jesus Christ; (4) this mercy affected woman's ethical position, but her physical condition remained unchanged; (5) her physical state has deteriorated as actual sins have added to each other; (6) yet she still has her will, with which to fight the predisposition to disease; (7) the duties of motherhood depend upon this will or strength of character; (8) she is required by God to submit to all the dangers of motherhood. It was with such things in mind as this and its bearing upon health that Aldous Huxley wrote of "that once very common over-simplification of the facts which consists in making God responsible for all imperfectly understood phenomena. Secondary causes are ignored and everything is referred back to the creator. No more wholesale reduction of diversity to identity is possible; and yet its effect is not immediately perceptible. Those who make the mistake of thinking in terms of a first cause are fated never to become men of science. But as they do not know what science is, they are not aware that they are losing anything."[14] The extent to which this almost classical original sin myth influences present-day Christians will vary a great deal, but to suppose that it is not influential would be to underestimate the prevailing complexity of religious attitudes as they bear upon the ethics of medical care.

To return to our ethical analysis, it should be clear that ectopic pregnancy is a pathological condition in which a fertilized egg is lodged in a fallopian tube and threatens death to both embryo and mother if it is permitted to continue. This means that in the surgical treatment of the condition, sterilization as well as abortion will be entailed: sterilization because a fallopian tube is cut out and hence future pregnancies to that extent are precluded, and abortion because the embryo is destroyed along with the tube. There is an amazingly detailed and argumentative discussion of this question by Father O'Malley in his *Ethics of Medical Homicide*. He is interested, of course, in defending the view that any aggression against an embryo from the time of conception to delivery is morally equivalent to manslaughter (when, that is to say, it is not directly intended as such; by legal logic it becomes murder when it is done for its own sake, or directly intended). This view is held because any embryo, even though it lacks any personal quality, is never-

[14] *Ends and Means*, London, 1948, p. 14.

theless, he maintains, a human being with all the human rights.

What, then, is to be done under these circumstances, when both mother and embryo will be destroyed if the pregnancy proceeds? The only life which actually can be saved, in the nature of the case, is the mother's. We could easily aggravate the ethical dilemma by reference to cases known to medical practice in which a double conception takes place ectopically, with one fertile ovum lodged in a fallopian tube and the other properly placed. In such a predicament there are three lives at stake, not merely two. To insist upon leaving the ectopic embryo "unaggressed" is to sacrifice not only the mother, but a brother or sister, according to the soul-infusion doctrine. Even if it were claimed that the mother knowingly undertakes all the risks of conception, so that an innocent third party may not be victimized to save her own life, what of the entirely innocent brother or sister unborn, to say nothing of those already born and dependent upon her for care and protection? The basic difficulty in the position arises, of course, from the soul-and-life idea which attributes personal status to a pre-personal organism and assigns it human rights, including the right to rites of salvation.

A question (number 35) about the surgical removal of an ectopic pregnancy was directed to the Congregation of the Holy Office for an official ruling. The reply, on March 5, 1902, was an unqualified prohibition. The answer read: "No, it is not lawful. Such a removal is a direct killing of the fetus and is therefore forbidden."[15] (Incidentally, the Grand Mufti's *fatwa* of January 25, 1937, also replied to a formal inquiry by saying that even therapeutic abortions are absolutely forbidden after the embryo has "quickened." This gives a mother from two to three months more grace or rescue-time than Catholics enjoy.)

[15] Quoted in P. A. Finney, *Moral Problems in Hospital Practice, op.cit.*, p. 135.

In keeping with this prohibition, Father Burke explains that "from the standpoint of moral science there may be a conflict of claims, but a conflict of rights is a contradiction."[16] A statement of this kind does not create a very knotty problem. As it stands, it is questionable, anyway. A "claim" is simply a right seeking recognition. Any claim which is not a right is either an innocent error or an attempt to cheat. Furthermore, to say that "a conflict of rights is a contradiction" is redundant, for "conflict" and "contradiction" are the same. What Father Burke really intends to say is, "There may be a conflict of claims, but there cannot be a conflict of rights." But this is absurd, because assuming the claims to be valid—that is to say, rightful claims—a conflict of claims *is* a conflict of rights. Therefore, all Father Burke can possibly assert is that there may be a *verbal* conflict of *verbal* claims, in which some are based upon right and some are not.

The real question raised by Father Burke's proposition—but hidden beneath some layers of language—is whether it is possible that rights *can* ever come into conflict, or contradict each other. Are rights, that is to say, in the nature of things both intrinsically and extrinsically exclusive, singular, unique? The right to live may be intrinsically unique and uncontingent, although even this is not in accord with the general maxim of moral theology that all rights are imperfect and therefore not always able to prevail. But even so they cease to be so extrinsically (*per accidens*) in such cases as ectopic pregnancy, where the mother's right to live is denied if the alleged right of the embryo to live is recognized. Therefore Father Burke can maintain his assertion that there cannot be a conflict of rights only by denying validity to the claim to life made on behalf of either the mother or the embryo! But this places him in a dilemma. If he denies that the right exists in either case, or if he so

[16] *Acute Cases of Moral Medicine, op.cit.,* p. 10.

acts as to violate the right of either, he then runs afoul of a basic assumption in his orthodox morality, namely, that all human beings have a right to life, predicated upon a Creationist theory of the soul. If, on the other hand, he remains loyal to the Creationist soul-doctrine he is compelled to repudiate his own proposition, since it asserts that there can be no conflict of rights! There is a way out for him, which is surely the sound one to take regardless of this particular question. This would be to deny that the right to life claimed for a fetus is valid, because a fetus is not a moral or personal being since it lacks freedom, self-determination, rationality, the ability to choose either means or ends, and knowledge of its circumstances. However, in Father Burke's case, this solution would only compound his difficulties with orthodoxy because of the official view (Proposition 34) that a life (*cum* "soul") is present from the very first moment of impregnation. It seems perfectly obvious that there is no ethical solution for him except to adopt, as we adopt, what Father Slater has called the materialist opinion that the embryo before birth is a portion of the mother, which may be excised if it threatens her life. Such action would be in accordance with the ruling of St. Thomas, as well as with the view of common sense and a humane perspective, that a part may be sacrificed for the sake of the whole. We might take note that Father Slater calls this a materialist view in spite of the fact that he himself refuses to permit spiritual and moral considerations to take precedence over the terms of brute physiology.

This whole question is of interest to historians because St. Thomas Aquinas, the Doctor of the Latin Church whose authority is probably greater than any other's in contemporary Catholicism, had ruled that one may protect one's life if necessary even at the expense of the aggressor's life (*Summa Theologica*, ii, ii, q.64, a.7). Just the same, the majority of moral theologians have fallen into line with Proposition

35; they prohibit any such effort to save the mother's life, *even though it is understood that the embryo will be destroyed anyway if it is allowed to proceed and destroy the mother.*[17]

We can easily imagine what most people would feel if a physician and a priest were to be sued in court after a woman had died under such circumstances. No case of this kind has ever reached court, and perhaps now it never will, because American and British theologians and clergy of the Catholic communion are rebelling against a position of such impossible dilemmas in value assignment and of such offense to their pastoral instincts. This rebellion takes the form of a reinterpretation of the papal doctrine. The *Homiletic and Pastoral Review* for October 1945 said, "Medical men today are quite commonly agreed that tubal pregnancy constitutes a pathological condition and is as much a threat to the mother's health as a cancerous uterus. The theologians of the last century who held that it is gravely sinful to remove an unruptured tube containing a living fetus, because such a procedure is direct killing, were right in their principle but wrong in their facts. . . . It is not direct but indirect killing."

How seriously are we to take this revision of the prior view? It amounts to saying that earlier moral theologians, and even the Holy Office itself, had failed by some strange myopia to see that their Rule of Double Effect applied to cases of treatment for ectopic pregnancy, that they failed to see that it applied as it does, for example, to hysterectomies during pregnancy when a maternal pathology is so serious that the operation cannot be postponed until the fetus is viable. How could they fail to detect so patent a parallel? To say they "were right in their principle but wrong in their facts" only muddies the waters, since the "facts," as

[17] An enlightening account is found in Walter Reaney's *Creation of the Soul,* New York, 1932.

153

distinct from moral intentions or motives, are objective medical conditions in no way altered since 1902, or likely to alter any faster than the feminine physiology can or may restructure itself. Father Davis attempts to save face by suggesting that the Holy Office had meant its prohibition to apply only to direct interference with an ectopic pregnancy, i.e., one which was aimed at ending the pregnancy rather than, presumably, saving the life of the mother. On any objective view, this would appear to be a reduction of the dilemma to an absurdity.[18]

Still another explanation is offered for the revision. This one recommends itself more strongly to ethical standards, but has only a minimum plausibility as far as "facts" are concerned. It frankly pleads previous ignorance. It is an attempt to explain that earlier theologians once underestimated the gravity of ectopic pregnancies ("their facts were wrong") *as a threat to the mother*, and for that reason they were justified in forbidding an operation because it was, as far as they could see, a direct attack on the embryo but not a direct act of self-defense for the mother. Now that they know that ectopics are a grave threat to the mother, they can invoke St. Thomas' rule that one may defend one's life by means which, if necessary, cost the aggressor's life. It is indirect, not direct, killing. It comes to this, that they do not *intend* to kill the fetus but only to save the mother's life, just as a policeman might not intend to kill a criminal, but only to defend his own life or a law-abiding citizen's. *Conserva me, Domine!* Thus there is a final resort to the ubiquitous Rule of Double Effect which we have seen brought to the rescue in other questions of morals and medicine. "Under certain circumstances we may be allowed to perform an action from which a two-fold result follows, one good, one evil. . . . If the good end or result of the action is desired (and the evil result is *not* desired), we may so act even though we know the evil

[18] *Moral and Pastoral Theology, op.cit.,* II, 175.

consequence will follow."[19] The rescue of the mother is intended; the destruction of the embryo is only an unfortunate by-product. This reasoning allows the theologians to persist in their natural-law claim combined with the soul-infusion theory, that an embryo is a real person, as real as the mother. At the same time it permits them to avoid a ruling which would be apt to land them before a bar of enlightened justice on a charge of murder when some grief-stricken husband or sectarian enemy could one day set up a test case. This is not an impossible turn of events, especially in view of strong religious animus and even bigotry in some quarters.

If we follow these lines, then, we see that the position at present in American Catholic hospitals comes down to the one described in the Catholic Hospital Association's directives. Readers should observe that the position does not bear out the popular false notion, quite commonly repeated for reasons of bigotry or political opposition to the Roman hierarchy, that Catholics "always choose the mother's life rather than the child's when a choice is necessary." The *Religious and Ethical Directives* clearly provide: "The *direct* killing of any innocent person, even at his own request, is always morally wrong. Any procedure whose sole immediate effect is the death of a human being is a *direct* killing. *Risk* to life and even the *indirect* taking of life are morally justifiable for proportionate reasons. (Life is taken *indirectly* when death is the unavoidable accompaniment or result of a procedure which is immediately directed to the attainment of some other purpose, e.g., the removal of a diseased organ.) Every unborn child must be considered as a human person, with all the rights of a human person, from the moment of conception." Among the indirect destructions of embryo children thus permitted are: "operations, treatments, and medications . . . of a proportionately serious pathological condition of the mother . . . even though they *indirectly*

[19] For the qualifying conditions, cf. above ch. 2, n. 38.

cause an abortion."[20] Added are Caesarean section, aspiration for hydrocephalus (of the fetal cranium for successful delivery, which may be fatal for the child), ectopic-pregnancy removal of an affected part of an ovary or tube, hysterectomy for a diseased uterus, premature delivery, radiation therapy. It seems fairly evident that a certain amount of uneasiness goes along with this kind of ethical reasoning, even though humane in its valuations, because it is tied dogmatically to the theory of the equality of mother and fetus. A telltale passage in Father Davis' work, having to do specifically with craniotomy, says open-endedly and contradictorily that in such cases "a Catholic doctor must give up the case, but he is not thereby precluded from telling those whom it may concern that other medical advice must be got, or rather may be got."[21] In any case, however we may prefer to explain this welcome shift of opinion, it marks a sound step forward from the older view of Father Thomas Slater that when a mother must choose between death or an abortion, she "must ask the doctor to prescribe some other remedy or palliative which will at least save her conscience if not her life."[22]

"Clear and Future Danger"

But now to tie all this necessary background directly into the question of sterilization, it should be clear that this reinterpretation of the dictum of 1902 allows a line of reasoning to permit preventive as well as curative sterilization. It works to that end because in cases where a disease or pathological condition requires treatment resulting in the dysfunctioning of an organ essential to procreation, the treatment is permissible on the basis of Double Effect. Will the rule, in fact, be extended to cover other cases calling for sterilization, cases more unilaterally preventive? The history

[20] *Op.cit.*, p. 4. Italics in the original.
[21] *Op.cit.*, II, 193.   [22] *Cases of Conscience, op.cit.*, I, 231.

of Catholic medical ethics suggests that the pressure of medical conscience and of rational morality will urge Roman Catholics on, however reluctantly, to expand their definition of pathologies widely enough to include even those human ills which are potential threats. If we had no right to obviate the dangers of some pathologies by sterilization, we would sometimes have to deny the sex life merely in order to avoid a fatal pregnancy or, for that matter, the pathology of a tragically defective child. This would mean that the unitive side of marriage would have to be made of none effect for the sake of a grim and irrational physical disorder. Meanwhile, we cannot help wondering how many mothers may have died uselessly and cruelly between 1902 and 1945 while the moral theologians were sticking fast to their theocratic absolutes; and, again, how many mothers may yet die in childbirth—or die in spirit, bearing personally hopeless children—while a double-effect defense is being found for preventive sterilization. In the end there must be some reasonable medical safeguard of personality and health in sterilization, even if it has to be put down as only an indirect attack on the magical untouchability of the natural body. Almost any ethical rationale is to be welcomed that will neutralize the physiological determinism of what has been called the doctrine of "the integrity of the body" in favor of a doctrine of the integrity of the personality.

For the present, then, the position is that sterilization is permitted by Catholic morals only as a right of self-defense in cases of what our Supreme Court calls "a clear and present danger." Catholic moralists will not allow any moral justification of sterilization as a preventive measure of self-defense, or as a practice in preventive medicine on a principle of "clear and *future* danger." It is ironic to observe that legal reasoning allows for justifiable homicide in cases where self-defense involving killing was planned ahead of the actual action, because the defender had to go armed or otherwise prepared, knowing that his life would be endangered by an enemy, and yet the moral theologians, for all their addiction to legalism, find no parallel between this and preventive sterilization. If they were to reply that the parallel breaks down because the defender does not kill his enemy *before* the enemy actually threatens his life, then in that case we could point out that there is a complete parallel in this regard between preventive sterilization and warfare, which has full justification both by civil lawyers and moral theologians! They will agree only that we may lawfully rid ourselves of an actual disease; but (such is the logic) where a future pregnancy would be fatal to the mother or to the child's personality, persons in such a case must either court death if they continue their sexual love or embrace chastity, regardless of its consequences for marriage, health, happiness, or any other value at stake.

Perhaps the simplest and briefest account of the Catholic position is found in the Encyclical Letter of Pius XI, *Casti Conubii* (On Chaste Marriage). This encyclical, given out on December 31, 1930, is the dogmatic basis of present-day doctrine and discipline on marriage and sex ethics. It says, among other things, that the body as nature provides it is to set the terms of physical well-being. "Christian doctrine establishes, and the light of human reason makes it most clear, that private individuals have no power over the members of their bodies than that which pertains to their natural ends; and they are not free to destroy or mutilate their members, or in any other way render themselves unfit for their natural functions, except where no other provision can be made for the good of the whole body." Apart from its explicit permission of curative sterilization, the encyclical offers two questionable sanctions for its opinion: first, that it is required by Christian doctrine, and, second, that human reason supports it. In addition, it declares that preventive sterilization is not a right of personal choice. Since it also denies, in another place, that the state has a right to offer or require sterilization, it follows that no human agency may do so. This is precisely the meaning of the assertion that we have no power (i.e., right of control) over our bodies in any other way "than that which pertains to their natural ends." Here again we are back to that counter-Reformation version of the Natural Law as something *physiologically* determined, which we have previously described as a denial of true morality, and as a submission to *fatality* and to physical (material) determinism. As we can see with special vividness in the ethics of medical care, this is a very profound and fundamental issue to be resolved in first principles.

The problem has been posed for us by scholars in fields other than moral theology. Benjamin Kidd, for example, who may not have been entirely uninfluenced by the moralists, used his *Social Evolution* to set out the same idea in sharp terms by contending that the invasion of all spheres of life by the intellect is fatal to the evolution of the human race. This theory is at least fully consistent with all theological attacks on rational human being and all forms, whether religious or not, of the revolt against reason. It is an outlook opposed to the belief that lies behind this book. To accept the anti-intellectual view would be, presumably, to say that organized religion has rendered an important service by keeping the rational faculty in check in matters of life, health, and death! But the checking power never seems to reach mate. As one moralist says ruefully, "Even our Catholic people are no longer accepting these truths. They are rationalizing about the Catholic teachings and standards."[23]

In the first place, there is no Christian doctrine which supports the prohibition of sterilization, for preventive reasons or for any reasons whatsoever. Indeed, there is no mention of the subject, explicitly or implicitly, in any Chris-

[23] F. M. Kirsch, *Sex Education and Training in Chastity*, New York, 1930, p. 454.

tian formulation anywhere, unless of course we accept the view that Pius himself provided the doctrine when he expressed the opinion. There is nothing of any kind like it in the Bible, in the creeds, in the findings of ecumenical councils. There was nothing on the subject even at Trent, or in any Lateran Council.

In the second place, there is certainly no open-and-shut case for the claim that "human reason makes it most clear," unless we are prepared to accept the idea that what nature usually does is "intended" by nature and ultimately, therefore, by God; and the further view that we may never lawfully question or qualify it. To rephrase our earlier analysis of this relentless moral theory—which on the principles we have adopted is a materialistic rather than a personalistic doctrine—we might say that it is only another, somewhat sophisticated version of primitive animism, a kind of ethical animism very much akin to what anthropologists call negative magic or tabu. It is nothing more than fear of nature, in modern dress and recondite theological garb!

The idea that sterilization to prevent conception is not a matter for individual control denies exactly what we have been pleading, namely, that moral responsibility requires such choices to be personal decisions rather than natural necessities. Later we shall speak of the pros and cons of eugenical sterilization by the state, to protect the social welfare and the social blood stream. But here we can say that whether or not the state may properly compel us to surrender our capacity to reproduce, or our capacity to become parents, there is no good ethical ground for denying us the right to choose this way of guaranteeing ourselves against death and personal tragedy as we fulfill our sexual needs, and of saving potentially defective children from being thrown into a life of misery and futility.

There is an assumption running throughout all that is said in behalf of our point of view, and it should be put clearly. It is that sexual love is inherently good, not evil; and expediently good, as a physical and psychological drive requiring normal satisfaction. It is further assumed that this drive may be rightfully satisfied, if it does not invade the rights of others, and if it does not destroy other values of equal or greater importance. Even the papal doctrine which insists that procreation is the primary purpose of marriage (and we can heartily agree with that relative scale, *mutatis mutandis*), allows for the secondary or proximate ends of marriage, viz., married love and the "remedy for concupiscence." As Koch-Preuss admits, we should regard matrimony "as a natural union, a moral society, and a sacramental association," and, "though the *sedatio concupiscentiae* and the propagation of the species are true purposes of Matrimony, yet its highest or principal object is the undivided community of life led by husband and wife."[24] This is what we have been saying in our use of the word "unitive" to describe the loving aspect of marriage, which is both a physical and a moral phenomenon. Indeed, every Roman theologian insists that sexual access is a matter of mutual right, a *debitum conjugale*, as plainly asserted by St. Paul.

It seems apparent, be it fully noted, that this right could be defended even on the physiological interpretation of natural law. If what nature intends is good, and if it is something with which we have no right to interfere, then clearly sexual love between marriage partners is as much a natural-law obligation as any consequential procreation. Love, in short, is as natural as parenthood. This is arguable, further-

[24] *Op.cit.*, v, 463-464. Cf. also T. L. Bouscaren, *Canon Law Digest, Suppl. through 1948*, Milwaukee, 1949, Decrees of the Holy Office on the Ends of Marriage, April 1, 1944, AAS36-103: "the primary end of marriage is the generation and education of children" and "the secondary ends are not essentially subordinate to the primary end, but are equally principal and independent." This seems to mean that marriage and coitus can aim at the unitive aspect of the marriage bond only if procreation is accepted and intended as the primary purpose, although it need not be so in every act of intercourse but only as an over-all attitude.

more, because it is clear that nature does not intend conception as a necessary part of sexual union, for we observe that it does not occur regularly or even in more than a negligible percentage of cases. But our plea is that this is not a highly ethical basis of justification. The merits and demerits of sexual union rest properly upon personal rights and values, not upon natural processes. We human beings are psychophysical creatures. Our spiritual and moral relationships, our responses to others, are most complete and genuine when they are voluntary surrenders and mutual commitments, including physical as well as spiritual comradeship. It is for this reason that we regard sexual love as good, not for any reason of naturalistic utility or physiological mystique. Therefore, when there is a good and sufficient cause to eliminate the possibility of reproduction against our rational will, in order responsibly to fulfill the obligations of love, we are more than justified morally in doing so.

Cure or Prevention, Either One

Thus far our attention has been concentrated upon the first of the three reasons for sterilization, the therapeutic reason, including both cure and prevention. That is because our concern, as the first chapter of this book explained, is "deliberately held to the level of personal morality, insofar as it may be realistically abstracted from social justice and public morality." Our attention is focussed upon "those moral issues which are, or in our opinion ought to be, regarded by general consent as matters of private choice and responsibility." This does not mean, of course, that personal choice and decision have a purely selfish, self-defensive, or individualistic frame of reference. While curative sterilization might conceivably be of that order, there are reasons other than mere self-defense for preventive sterilization or choosing to foreclose reproduction. In preventive sterilization there is at stake the whole matter of the potential child's rights to health of mind and body. Thus the preventive side of therapeutic sterilization coincides immediately with eugenic sterilization, the second form of the practice mentioned at the opening of this chapter.

If the foremost concern of the Christian ethic, for example, is (as it could be shown to be) with personality, then we are under great obligation to consider how our moral choices affect not only ourselves but others. If on the other hand we were to hold that the foremost concern of the Christian ethic is with souls and that the soul is a supernatural something, *ein metaphysisches etwas*, entirely independent of and unconditioned by personality, and "not made for the earth and time but for heaven and eternity," then we should indeed take a different view of the ethics of sterilization. But our view is just the opposite; we put the priority on personality, and frankly view with skepticism the claim for a soul as an entity apart from life and personal being. Furthermore, we regard personality as only partly a biological phenomenon, and for the rest a social or cultural creation. Human persons are, in the very nature of personal existence, members of the community. A man is, as Aristotle said, a *zoon politikon*, a social being, and St. Thomas followed him strictly on that score. Indeed, our capacity to be or to become persons is realized within and by means of our social relations. We cannot be persons, or moral beings, in isolation from the lives of others, for our responsibility is exercised in response to other moral beings, other people with rights and duties as valid and real as our own. Therefore we are always under obligation morally to recognize the rule of the innocent third party, i.e., that we may not solve conflicts of interest at the expense of the innocent person who may be or could be involved and victimized by our decisions.

The fact is that sex is precisely the physical nexus of mankind, as speech is the cultural nexus. When this concept is related to sterilization, it means that the claims of parent-hood lose their validity if our knowledge of the medical facts reveals that children born to us will inherit grave diseases or defects, especially if we have at our command a means to prevent such tragedies. This follows, just as logically as the belief that we have no valid claim to the right to speak or otherwise communicate with our fellow men if what we produce is evil or destructive or false. We must wholly and passionately reject the view expressed by Father Slater that "to exist even with a taint is better than not to exist at all," and that "the calendar of Christian saints would be much shorter, nay, it would be robbed of some of its most glorious names, if all the degenerates were to be removed from it."[25] Such a statement is reminiscent of St. Anselm's medieval opinion, expressed in connection with his ransom theory of the Atonement doctrine, that God creates souls in order to save them, thus replacing the fallen angels, whose defection had reduced the size of the heavenly choir to much less than the divine taste required! The encyclical of Pius XI al-ready quoted (p. 158) says the same thing, and we are left to suppose that an idiot, cut off from personal growth and self-realization, is as good a candidate for the post-mortem life (or choir) as a normal person.

We are drawn into the opposite direction by the principles of personal worth. We cannot escape from the conviction that it is a grave wrong and a betrayal of the Christian conception of personality, as well as against a rational con-science, to allow stunted and defective lives to be propagated when the means are available in medicine to prevent it. It would seem blasphemous to assert that God wills or pur-poses that defective children should be born. Let the theolo-gians, in their speculative systems based on first causes, solve in some other way the problem of conflict between God's goodness and the fact of evil in the genes and chromosomes!

[25] "Eugenics and Moral Theology," in *Questions*, *op.cit.*, pp. 252-271.

Normal people are responsible, and that responsibility includes bringing new lives into the world. "To put the responsibility upon God when such lives are defective is a wilful refusal or inability to face the facts."[26] It compounds the error of animism and tabu with a mechanistic theodicy in which God assumes the appearance of a Moloch playing a game of profit and loss, with people being manipulated as pawns instead of being met as persons in a divine-human encounter. More even than this, it is a self-regarding claim of unique interest when it is used to make a biological right absolute and to deny a person his right to sacrifice himself, or his desire of posterity, for the good of the community. "Greater love than this hath no man": to repudiate this is to repudiate the altruism of the Christian ethic. It is possible, given the tragic circumstances, that we could literally as well as figuratively "make ourselves eunuchs for the kingdom of heaven's sake."

With all this in mind, how can we come to any other conclusion than that we are on good moral ground if we choose, by the canons of freedom and knowledge, to employ sterilization for reasons of cure or prevention, either one? All of this means, if it is sound, that personally we are justified in choosing and freely seeking sterilization as an ethical form of medical care. But there still remains the problem of whether we may rightfully be compelled, by the state or some other public authority, to undergo sterilization in the interest of the public welfare. Eugenic motives are legitimate—indeed, they are obligatory—in the field of personal morality. But what about social morality and social control? The second and third of the causes advanced for sterilization—the eugenic and punitive—fall into this context of social ethics. Before closing this chapter, we ought

[26] J. P. Hinton and J. E. Calcutt, *Sterilization: A Christian Approach.* London, 1935, p. 151. This volume marshals a case for sterilization in terms of social policy, but has little to say on the ethics of its personal use.

to make just one or two observations on this score, if only because the eugenic and punitive policies are so inevitably related to personal integrity.

Up to the present, 32 of the 48 states have passed sterilization laws, and they have been adopted also in Puerto Rico. Puerto Rico is a Catholic island in which contraceptive laws have also been passed by the insular legislature, without *intransigeant* opposition from the church. Three states (New York, Alabama, and Washington) have since repealed or inactivated their laws because of legal technicalities, but not for any asserted reasons of injustice or abuse. By 1952 more than 53,000 official operations had been performed under these laws. In Europe similar legislation is operative in Denmark, Esthonia, Germany, Norway, Sweden, the Soviet Union, and Switzerland. Japan adopted a law in 1948. In the United States, 23 states (and Puerto Rico) provide for compulsory sterilization after hearings before competent boards of control, 3 more have laws which are both compulsory and voluntary, and 2 others provide for only voluntary sterilization. Only Minnesota and Vermont, like Denmark, have a purely voluntary law. Massachusetts, as we might expect, has none at all; but in Connecticut, where contraceptive medicine is banned, there is nevertheless a sterilization law, of, incidentally, the compulsory kind. The constitutionality of these laws when they are compulsory is based upon the ethical reasoning to be found in such Supreme Court decisions as the one written by Justice Oliver Wendell Holmes in 1927, in which he said, "The principle that sustains compulsory vaccination is broad enough to cover cutting the Fallopian tubes (Jacobsen *v.* Massachusetts, 197 U.S. 11). Three generations of imbeciles are enough."[27]

Up to now we have seen strong reasons for voluntary sterilizations, but are there equally strong ones for compulsory sterilization, in cases where prospective parents are

[27] *Buck v. Bell, Superintendent,* U.S. Reports, 274.200.

incapable of or indifferent to responsible choice? Many serious investigators draw the line at governmental fiat. When the American Neurological Association had a committee study the problems of sterilization law, its chairman, Dr. Abraham Myerson of Boston, reported: "Any law concerning sterilization passed in the United States should be voluntary and regulatory rather than compulsory." It seems entirely legitimate to avail oneself of this distinction between mandatory and permissive law, as we saw in the case of contraceptive birth control. This is done in the recent Brock report of the British government, which says that sterilization should be a privilege, not an obligation or a penalty. Father Davis, in a conventional Catholic condemnation of compulsory sterilization, alleges that the "dominant motive, therefore, of those who recommend the eugenical sterilization of the unfit is the benefit of the State."[28] This is again the objection based upon abuse. It has in mind such perversions as the genocidal Nazi laws of the Third Reich in January 1933. The objection disregards *abusus non tollit usum*. It depends upon a dangerous, however unintentional, and authoritarian identification by such moralists of the state with society or the community of which the state apparatus is only a creature, only one agent and institution. At bottom, the right of society to be clean and safe, and the right of every child to be sound of mind and body, are the things at stake in the argument for compulsory sterilization. Developing research has tended to show that many diseases—such as renal calculus, nephritis, uterine cancer, and certain toxemias of pregnancy—are not only infective or environmental in origin but may be due to an hereditary vulnerability as well. It is for this reason that an observer such as E. A. Hooton complains that medical education ordinarily ignores genetics, and he insists that "it

---

[28] *Op.cit.*, II, 157.

is high time pathologists and geneticists [began to] sit up and take notice."[29]

It is impossible to see how the principle of social justice—at least on any very profound view of it—can be satisfied if the community may not defend itself, and is forced to permit the continued procreation of feeble-minded or hereditarily diseased children. Sterilization in such cases is not solely a matter of commutative justice (or personal control), but also of distributive justice (or state control). If it is argued that the segregation of such creatures is an alternative to sterilization, then our reproach will be that something more than personal values are being protected by that argument. There is too much clinical or empirical evidence to be seen in institutions for the feeble-minded, for example, to believe for a minute that personal integrity is being or could be realized in such places. The argument that all people, regardless of their stature as persons or their capacity to become persons, have a natural-law right to their procreative faculties and that we may not rightfully take them away, is just as fully circumvented by segregation as by sterilization. In the natural order it is an observable rule that what does not function dies, and the parallel principle in ethics is that rights which are denied their exercise are dead, although not necessarily invalidated. There is no difference between compulsory sterilization and compulsory segregation. The latter quite effectively takes away sexual freedom and destroys procreation. This is so obvious that one finds it hard to avoid seeing the arbitrary and obstructive character of an outlook which will deny society all right to protect itself, except by isolating already limited creatures, and at the same time condemns children, as far as prevenient wisdom is concerned, to enter upon a tragic and frustrated existence in a world they cannot understand

[29] "Human Heredity," address to the College of Physicians, Philadelphia, Apr 24, 1942.

or cope with. Whether this is to provide God with another soul to save, or for some other soteriological reason, seems, to say the least, to be an astounding predicate in its consequences.

The punitive reason for sterilization, likewise repudiated by most moral theologians, offers very little perplexity of conscience. It is commonly said that penal justice has three ends or purposes: (1) vindication of the law (its vindictive aspect); (2) reformation of the criminal; and (3) restraint of the criminal. Unless we accept the Old Testament *lex talionis*—the law of "an eye for an eye and a tooth for a tooth"—it seems that there is no moral gain to be had in vindictive punishment by means of sterilization. Nor is it at all easy to see how sterilization will reform a criminal of low intelligence, perhaps one who is an habitual sex offender. The evidence of psychiatric medicine and of recidivism in court records points to an opposite conclusion. This leaves only one valid reason for punitive sterilization, namely, restraint. To justify restraining criminals from procreating by sterilization takes us right back ethically over the ground we covered in discussing preventive sterilization. The ethics of compulsory treatment where irresponsibility or criminal indifference are present raises the same ethical questions we found there. If, as a matter of social justice, it may sometimes be necessary to deprive a criminal—say a rapist—of the power of procreation, then punitive sterilization for the sake of restraint is ethically sound.

Nature or Nurture?

In dealing with the ethics of sterilization as a method of medical care and treatment, we have seen that the opposition in formal ethics comes from Catholic moralists in a systematic way. But as in other matters, theirs is not the only opposition; it is only more uniform and more carefully reasoned. The opposition stems from an unmistakable reluctance to accept the principles of human freedom and human knowledge. Back of this attitude there often lies a false and inhuman doctrine about natural law. As Dean Inge has said, "it is disquieting for Christians to have to admit that the growth of humanity, in the sense of humaneness, does not owe much to the churches."[30] It was this aspect of practical humanitarianism which so deeply troubled the American pioneer of sterilization (and the telephone!), Alexander Graham Bell. Like his, our position has been opposed to naturalism in ethics, which we have claimed is primitive and animistic. It could be said that this has been a debate of nature versus nurture, with our pleading on the side of nurture. But our view is against nature only in the sense that it subordinates physical nature to human nature. We cannot submit to physiology and its irrational patterns without abdicating our moral status. Walt Whitman's talk about the "divine average" of humanity is a strange form of mysticism when seen in the perspective of social biology and human choice. After all, we can say with good reason that Gresham's law—that bad money tends to drive out good—can operate in genetics too! As S. J. Holmes puts it, "We cannot raise a fine crop of human beings without attending to *both* nature and nurture."[31] Spiritual stature comes with the nurture. Indeed, nurture of personal responsibility means precisely that nature is being qualified by the spirit and the "sapiens" in *homo sapiens*.

For many Christian lay people forbidden to consider sterilization, who may feel the weight of our ethical analysis, there is a word of hope and comfort, and we offer it only half in jest. Repentance in Christian doctrine is supposed to be a high virtue as well as the gateway to a larger life. Why not, then, if unhappy circumstances require it, obey the moral claims of sterilization, and then repent, that is, be

[30] *Christian Ethics and Modern Problems*, New York, 1930, p. 281.
[31] *Life and Morals*, New York, 1948, p. 207.

sorry, as any sensible person would be anyway! *The American Ecclesiastical Review* says that a sterilized person, if repentant, may resume his or her marriage rights without sinning.[32] Surely we ought to be able to find some humane way of dealing with the natural law by using a double team of the theology of penitence and the Rule of Double Effect! After all, ecclesiastical princes have managed somehow to justify the sterilization of boys in order to provide *soprani falsetti* voices for the Sistine choirs of Rome.[33] If sterilization can be justified for the sake of an earthly choir and heavenly music, surely we can find a way to justify it for human growth and personality and the harmony of physical well-being. It might be along lines of this sort, somehow, that the churches can free themselves of such bitter observations as the Gloomy Dean's that "churches, after all, are secular institutions in which the half-educated cater for the half-converted."[34] Otherwise, those branches of the Christian church which cling to their ethically primitive animism will indeed become *vox clamantis in deserto.*

[32] 99.563, Dec. 1938.

[33] Practiced as early as Sylvester I (A.D. 314-335) and not stopped until Leo XIII in 1884. Cf. the statement of Benedict XIV (1740-1758) *De Syn. Dioec.* I.xi, c.7, n.3, in J.-P. Migne, *Theologiae Cursus Completus*, Montrouge, 1841, p. 1286, disapproving but accepting the custom.

[34] W. R. Inge, *Talks in a Free Country*, London, 1943, p. 49.

CHAPTER SIX

EUTHANASIA: OUR RIGHT TO DIE

Where Is the Sting of Death?

EUTHANASIA, the deliberate easing into death of a patient suffering from a painful and fatal disease, has long been a troubling problem of conscience in medical care. For us in the Western world the problem arises, *pro forma*, out of a logical contradiction at the heart of the Hippocratic Oath. Our physicians all subscribe to that oath as the standard of their professional ethics. The contradiction is there because the oath promises two things: first, to relieve suffering, and second, to prolong and protect life. When the patient is in the grip of an agonizing and fatal disease, these two promises are incompatible. Two duties come into conflict. To prolong life is to violate the promise to relieve pain. To relieve the pain is to violate the promise to prolong and protect life.

Ordinarily an attempt is made to escape the dilemma by relieving the pain with an analgesic that does not induce death. But this attempt to evade the issue fails in many cases for the simple reason that the law of diminishing returns operates in narcosis. Patients grow semi-immune to its effects, for example in some forms of osteomyelitis, and a dose which first produces four hours of relief soon gives only three, then two, then almost none. The dilemma still stands: the choice between euthanasia or suffering. Euthanasia may be described, in its broadest terms, as a "theory that in certain circumstances, when owing to disease, senility or the like, a person's life has permanently ceased to be either agreeable or useful, the sufferer should be painlessly killed, either by himself or by another."[1] More simply, we may call euthanasia merciful release from incurable suffering.

---

[1] H. J. Rose, "Euthanasia," *Eneyc. of Rel. and Ethics*, v, 598-601.

Our task in this book is to put the practice under examination in its strictly medical form, carefully limiting ourselves to cases in which the patient himself chooses euthanasia and the physician advises against any reasonable hope of recovery or of relief by other means. Yet even in so narrowly defined an application as this, there are conscientious objections, of the sort applied to broader concepts or usages. In the first place it is claimed that the practice of euthanasia might be taken as an encouragement of suicide or of the wholesale murder of the aged and infirm. Again, weak or unbalanced people may more easily throw away their lives if medical euthanasia has approval. Still another objection raised is that the practice would raise grave problems for the public authority. Government would have to overcome the resistance of time-honored religious beliefs, the universal feeling that human life is too sacred to be tampered with, and the problem of giving euthanasia legal endorsement as another form of justifiable homicide. All of this could lead to an appalling increase of crimes such as infanticide and geronticide. In short, in this problem as in others which we have been analyzing there is a common tendency to cry abuse and to ignore *abusus non tollit usum.*

Prudential and expedient objections to euthanasia quickly jump to mind among many people confronted with the issue. There are few, presumably, who would not be moved by such protests as this one from the *Linacre Quarterly*: "Legalized euthanasia would be a confession of despair in the medical profession; it would be the denial of hope for further progress against presently incurable maladies. It would destroy all confidence in physicians, and introduce a reign of terror. . . . [Patients] would turn in dread from the man on whose wall the Hippocratic Oath proclaims, 'If any shall ask of me a drug to produce death I will not give it, nor will I suggest such counsel.' "[2]

[2] Hilary R. Werts, S.J., in April, 1947, 19.2, p. 33.

However, it is the objection that euthanasia is inherently wrong, that the disposition of life is too sacred to be entrusted to human control, which calls for our closest analysis. As in preceding chapters, here too we shall be dealing with the *personal* dimensions of morality in medical care. The social ethics of medical care, as it is posed to conscience by proposals to use euthanasia for eugenic reasons, population control, and the like, have to be left for another time and place.

Not infrequently the newspapers carry stories of the crime of a spouse, or a member of the family or a friend, of a hopelessly stricken and relentlessly tortured victim of, let us say, advanced cancer. Desperate people will sometimes take the law into their own hands and administer some lethal dose to end it all. Sometimes the euthanasiast then commits suicide, thus making two deaths instead of one. Sometimes he is tried for murder in a court of law, amid great scandal and notoriety. But even if he is caught and indicted, the judgment never ends in conviction, perhaps because the legalism of the charge can never stand up in the tested conscience of a sympathetic jury.

For the sake of avoiding offense to any contemporaries, we might turn to literary history for a typical example of our problem. Jonathan Swift, the satirist and Irish clergyman, after a life of highly creative letters ended it all in a horrible and degrading death. It was a death degrading to himself and to those close to him. His mind crumbled to pieces. It took him eight years to die while his brain rotted. He read the third chapter of Job on his birthday as long as he could see. "And Job spake, and said, Let the day perish when I was born, and the night in which it was said, There is a man child conceived." The pain in Swift's eye was so acute that it took five men to hold him down, to keep him from tearing out his eye with his own hands. For the last three years he sat and drooled. Knives had to be kept entirely out of his reach. When the end came, finally, his fits of convulsion lasted thirty-six hours.[3] Now, whatever may be the theological meaning of St. Paul's question, "O death, where is thy sting?"[4] the moral meaning—in a word, the evil—of a death like that is only too plain.

We can imagine the almost daily scene preceding Swift's death. (Some will say we should not imagine such things, that it is not fair to appeal to emotion. Many good people cannot willingly accept the horrendous aspects of reality as a factor of reasoning, especially when reality cuts across their customs and commitments. The relative success with which we have repressed the reality of atomic warfare and its dreadful prospects is an example on a wider scale.) We can easily conceive of Dean Swift grabbing wildly, madly, for a knife or a deadly drug. He was *demoralized*, without a vestige of true self-possession left in him. He wanted to commit what the law calls suicide and what vitalistic ethics calls sin. Standing by was some good doctor of physick, trembling with sympathy and frustration. Secretly, perhaps, he wanted to commit what the law calls murder. Both had full knowledge of the way out, which is half the foundation of moral integrity, but unlike his patient the physician felt he had no freedom to act, which is the other half of moral integrity. And so, meanwhile, necessity, blind and unmoral, irrational physiology and pathology, made the decision. It was in reality no decision at all, no moral behavior in the least, unless submission to physical ruin and spiritual disorganization can be called a decision and a moral choice. For let us not forget that in such tragic affairs there is a moral destruction, a spiritual disorder, as well as a physical degeneration. As Swift himself wrote to his niece fully five years before the end: "I am so stupid and confounded that I cannot express the mortification I am under both of body and soul."[5]

[3] Virginia Moore, *Ho for Heaven*, New York, 1946, pp. 180-182.
[4] I Cor. 15:55.
[5] Quoted by Richard Garnett, "Jonathan Swift" in *Encyc. Brit.*, 11th ed.

The story of this man's death points us directly to the broad problem of suicide, as well as to the more particular problem of euthanasia. We get a glimpse of this paradox in our present customary morality, that it sometimes condemns us to live or, to put it another way, destroys our moral being for the sake of just *being*. This aspect of suicide makes it important for us to distinguish from the outset between voluntary and involuntary euthanasia. They are by no means the same, either in policy or ethical meaning. Those who condemn euthanasia of both kinds would call the involuntary form murder and the voluntary form a compounded crime of murder and suicide if administered by the physician, and suicide alone if administered by the patient himself. As far as voluntary euthanasia goes, it is impossible to separate it from suicide as a moral category; it is, indeed, a form of suicide. In a very proper sense, the case for medical euthanasia depends upon the case for the righteousness of suicide, given the necessary circumstances. And the justification of its administration by an attending physician is therefore dependent upon it too, under the time-honored rule that what one may lawfully do another may help him to do.

"Untouchability"

Felo de se—literally, being a criminal toward oneself, but in common usage meaning to take one's own life—is, of course, as old as mankind and human pain. This is true in spite of the valid generalization that the wish to live is among the strongest instinctual drives in the higher animals, including men. It is true regardless of the reasons we may offer, psychological or otherwise, to explain the frequent occurrence of exceptions to the rule. Some savage tribes laugh at suicide; some practice it freely. Others believe it earns a terrible punishment in the next world, and, like some Christian churches, deny all suicides a religious burial. Many of the Eastern religions allow it without censure, and even encourage it ceremonially. We find this to be true in the ancient Aztec and Inca cultures, but also more recently in the traditional Hindu practice of *suttee*, in which a widow throws herself onto the funeral pyre alongside her husband's body. The Japanese, of Buddhist and Shinto belief, have committed *hara-kiri* after losing face or suffering loss of prestige, or as a remarkably unaggressive reply to insult, as compared, for example, to the dueling code in Western manners. The Greeks and Romans were divided in their opinions about suicide, and therefore about euthanasia. If there were those among them who condemned it rigidly and absolutely, they were few and not given to publishing their views. Some moralists repudiated it as a general practice. For example, Pythagoras, Plato, and Aristotle held that suicide was a crime against the community because it robbed society of a resource, and Plato added that it was a like crime against God. But all of these were willing to justify suicide in cases calling for a merciful death.[6] Stoics usually, but not always, approved of suicide. Cicero, for example, condemned it, whereas Seneca praised it. Epictetus sided with Seneca. But they *all* favored euthanasia. Valerius Maximus said that magistrates at Marseilles kept a supply of poison on hand for those who could convince them that there was good reason for them to die.

The Semitic religions, Judaism and Mohammedanism, were opposed consistently to suicide. Being more Oriental than the Hellenic doctrines, they tended to regard physiological life as sacrosanct and untouchable, and they also tended to be more materialistic in their conception of the vital principle, so that the Jews located life in the blood— and thus their rules about kosher meat. The Christians, as a Jewish sect, went even further with a belief in physical or

[6] Plato, *Laws*, IX, 873 C; Aristotle, *Politics*, 1335 b, 19ff.; for Pythagoras, cf. Cicero, *Cato Major* 20 (72 sq.) and *De Officiis*, i.31 (112).

bodily resurrection to eternal life. Nevertheless, neither the Bible nor the Koran actually set forth an explicit condemnation of suicide, in any form, even though Jewish and Moslem commentators generally were against it. There is a tradition that Mohammed himself refused to bury a suicide. Certainly under the Hebrew influence, which put a heavier stamp of approval and meaning upon historical existence, being this-worldly rather than other-worldly, there was little philosophical ground in the West for the *tedium vitae* of Hinduism. A practice such as *suttee* was simply not within its ideological orbit.

The early Christians, like Chrysostom, followed the rabbis for the most part. A great many of the patristic writers allowed for suicide in certain forms, however, usually to achieve martyrdom, to avoid apostasy, or to retain the crown of virginity. Thus Lactantius declared that it is wicked to bring death upon oneself voluntarily, unless one was "expecting all torture and death" at the hands of the pagan persecutors.[7] Unfortunately for the precedent moralists he never bothered to apply his logic about torture and death to incurable diseases.

But once Christianity and the Roman government joined forces, the authority permitting suicide in persecution was withdrawn. We find St. Jerome allowing it only as a defense of chastity.[8] And then St. Augustine swept away even that exception by announcing that chastity, after all, is a virtue of the soul rather than of the body, so that physical violation did not touch it. St. Augustine cast aside the observation that the Scriptures nowhere condemned suicide, and that they even reported without comment or condemnation the suicides of Ahithophel by hanging, Zimri by fire, Abimelech by sword, Samson by crushing, and Saul by sword. He said with fine simplicity that the Scriptures nowhere *authorized*

---

[7] *Divinae institutiones*, vi.17.
[8] *Commentarii in Jonam*, i.12.

us to eliminate ourselves.[9] This became the conventional Christian position, and St. Thomas Aquinas gave it its classical form in the saying, "Suicide is the most fatal of sins, because it cannot be repented of."[10] We find that Christian burial was denied to suicides as early as A.D. 563.[11] The Roman Church to this day, by canonical prohibition, refuses to bury a suicide.

Unlike Judaism and Catholicism, Protestantism does not unanimously outlaw suicide, although various bodies will from time to time condemn euthanasia, or call it into question. As recently as 1951 the General Assembly of the Presbyterian Church in the U.S.A. resolved that suicide is contrary to the Sixth Commandment. In the Renaissance the reverence of West Europeans for the Greeks and Romans led to some easing of the old prohibition of suicide, especially in favor of euthanasia, but this was in tension with the Semitic attitude in Christianity. Here and there, occasionally, but almost always outside the Roman jurisdiction, there were testimonies to a new attitude. Thomas More, whose Utopia included euthanasia, was reflecting a new evaluation of human worth and integrity.[12] Lord Francis Bacon in his *New Atlantis* said, "I esteem it the office of a physician not only to restore the health, but to mitigate pains and dolors; and not only when such mitigation may conduce to recovery, but when it may serve to make a fair and easy passage." It was more commonly the Protestant and humanist moralists who relaxed the old prohibition. A typical effort was made in a little book called *Biathanatos* by John Donne, the Anglican priest and poet, dean of St. Paul's, a book which he described on the title page as a "Declaration of that paradoxe, or thesis, that Self-homicide is not so naturally sin, that it may never be otherwise."[13]

[9] *De civitate dei*, i.16 sq.   [10] *Summa Theologica*, ii.-ii 64.5.3.
[11] Westermarck, *Christianity and Morals, op.cit.*, p. 254.
[12] *Utopia*, ii, viii, "Of bondemen, sicke persons etc."
[13] London, 1648.

John Donne was a man who knew what death could be, because he lived for so long in its shadow and marked its many turns. His lines will always live, "Send not to ask for whom the bell tolls; it tolls for thee."[14] It is possible, but not certain, that Jeremy Taylor's *Holy Dying* favored merciful release in somewhat equivocal terms. At any rate, even theologians were beginning to doubt that Hamlet was altogether correct in supposing that "the everlasting" had "fixed his canon 'gainst self-slaughter."

The common civil law has always followed the line of the moral theologians. For centuries suicides were refused last rites by the church and their property impounded by the state. The English law about staking out a suicide's body at the crossroads—a law due partly to Christian theory and partly to fear of ghosts—was not abolished until the reign of George IV. The first really sharp break came with the French Revolution, when France abolished her old laws about suicide, especially the more grotesque priestly features. Then other Continental countries began to follow suit. The churches had held to their absolute prohibition, except for sporadic practices like that of the seventeenth-century people of Brittany, who allowed an incurable sufferer to appeal to the parish priest for the Holy Stone. The family gathered, the patient received the viaticum and last rites, and the oldest living relative raised the heavy stone above the patient's head and let it fall.

England moved very slowly in the matter, thus being very English about it! Her legal prohibition of suicide in any form continued in force, even though there were still a hundred and fifty crimes punishable by death, but it became the custom of juries to presume "absence of mind" or mental derangement in those who attempted or succeeded at *felo de se*. The standard verdicts of "suicide while of unsound mind" or "temporary insanity" had two motives:

[14] *Sermon on the Bells.*

to remove any stigma from the memory of the deceased, and to prevent confiscation by the state of his property as a post-mortem punishment. As Jeremy Bentham said in his *Principles of Penal Law*, this evasion of the issue by juries meant that perjury became the penance with which they prevented an outrage on humanity. Perhaps, among moralists, the utilitarians like Bentham have been most favorable to the notion of justifiable homicide. When Bentham died, consistent to the last, he asked his doctor to "minimize pain" with his dying breath. The last of the great English philosophers to pay any attention to the old theological arguments, even by way of opposing them, was David Hume in his essay *On Suicide* in 1777.[15] Hume crystallized the issue for medical ethics with his formulation that if our shortening lives interferes with Providence, medical services are already interfering by lengthening them.

It may be worth while to recall that the early church condemned the taking of life in military service, and yet it finally consented to it when a political concordat became a strong enough inducement.[16] It also condemned capital punishment as the taking of life, insisting that life is the sole property of God and at his sole disposition, and yet finally agreed to it when the church and state became partners. This double standard is now a part of our established mores or customary morality. We are, by some strange habit of mind and heart, willing to impose death but unwilling to permit it: we will justify humanly contrived death when it violates the human integrity of its victims, but we condemn it when it is an intelligent voluntary decision. If death is not inevitable anyway, not desired by the subject, and not merciful, it is righteous! If it is happening anyway and is freely embraced and merciful, then it is wrong! In the Roman communion the prohibition of suicide is presupposed in

[15] *Essays and Treatises*. London, 1777.
[16] C. J. Cadoux, *The Early Christian Attitude to War*, London, 1919, pp. 96-160.

certain canonical regulations.[17] There is, however, no clear
and certain united front of opinion among Catholic moralists on *medical* euthanasia, apparently because of the
difficulties created by the death-inducing effects of anesthesia.
Thus Father Davis says if the drugs "shorten life . . .
euthanasia is murder, and indefensible."[18] But Koch-Preuss
says, "To hasten death artificially . . . *can be regarded as
permissible* only if the drugs employed *for this purpose* do
not entirely deprive the sufferer of consciousness."[19] Thus it
becomes clear that the concern of this moralist is not with
life qua life and its sacrosanctity, but with *consciousness,*
which is needed for the patient's cooperation in last rites.
And of course there is the further complication or confusion of an opinion like St. Alphonsus Liguori's that a man
would be justified in taking his own life to escape death
in a more painful form, e.g., by leaping from a window to
get out of a burning building.[20] Yet even St. Alphonsus'
opinion is not left without doubt. Lehmkuhl goes only so
far as to say that if a man is condemned by the state to die
at his own hand, as in Socrates' case, he would be allowed
to obey, although not obliged to since it could be defended
as a probable opinion that the act is forbidden by natural
law.[21] We are left, therefore, to suppose that we may not
choose to die decently instead of living indecently, but if
we are to die horribly—through a necessity imposed upon
us by a pathology or some other tragic cause—then we are
free to exercise a preference between the kind of horror we
undergo, just so we are sure to be fully conscious of our

[17] *Codex Iuris Can.,* 1240, 1, n. 3.

[18] *Op.cit.,* II, 195.

[19] *Op.cit.,* III, 91. Italics added.

[20] *Op.cit.,* III, n. 367. Liguori permits such actions on the principle of double
effect, saying that they must be adapted to escape even though they will not
succeed: *Theologia Moralis,* III, n. 367. "Licet vero se *indirecte* occidere: puta,
si quis se ejiciat per fenestram, ut effugiat incendium; praesertim si adsit aliqua
spes mortem evandendi."

[21] *Theologica moralis,* 11th ed., 1.404.

suffering! As yet mercy has failed to exert an influence upon many Christians equal to the pull or pressure of power.

This is still the case among Christian moralists generally, and even among some pagan moralists. They are ready to justify the taking of the lives of others but balk at any reason for taking their own! A commission of American Protestants recently concluded that the mass extermination of civilians by atom-bomb blasts can be "just," although many of the members of the commission would hesitate to agree that fatal suffering could be ended righteously for one of the victims burned and charred externally and internally, not even as a response to the victim's plea. But the beatitude "Blessed are the merciful, for they shall obtain mercy" is still in the New Testament, as a part of the divine law. And the New Testament is still in the churches, and the churches are still based for authority on the New Testament. Therefore, as they have changed in some other things, so they may change in this too.[22] Some may come to feel that the divine law takes priority. Among many Christians the line of distinction between natural and divine often appears to be blurred or even erased, with no preference as to the claims of nature and the claims of grace. But most certainly if there is any provision in the divine law or revealed will of God as found in the Bible, it is the fifth beatitude calling for mercy. This is, ethically speaking, a great leap from the *talion* of the Semitic code and the ruthlessness of nature. Mercy cannot by any stretch of the imagination be found to be a plausible statistical average of events or behavior in the natural creation. Natural reason applied to nature could

[22] The latest pronouncement of a church body came from the Episcopal Church in 1952. Noting "a growing movement to legalize the practice of Euthanasia," it was resolved that "the members of the General Convention of the Protestant Episcopal Church place themselves in opposition to the legalizing of the practice of Euthanasia, under any circumstances whatsoever." *Journal of the General Convention of the Protestant Episcopal Church*, 1952, p. 216. It should be noted that the resolution actually only opposes making euthanasia legal: it does not oppose the practice. This may be due to poor drafting, and not intentional.

never deduce that mercy is "intended" or "in the mind" of the created physical order. Mercy is a value or virtue born of personal growth and moral stature, a thing of the spirit altogether. By itself nature cannot produce it.

Law and Malice

The present-day legal status of euthanasia, the one form of taking life with which we are concerned in medical morals, is neither ethically clear nor satisfactory to conscience. This is the situation everywhere in the Western world, not only in our own country but in Latin America and Europe, including Soviet Russia. The law of murder fails to take any account of the physical and mental, and hence of the spiritual, condition of the victim or subject of the murder action. Suicide is always a legal felony. As moralists, those who would justify euthanasia have to ask the lawyers and lawmakers to recognize it as justifiable homicide rather than a felony, whether it is merciful death self-administered by the patient, with medical advice, or administered by the physician. There is, at bottom, no real moral difference between self-administered euthanasia and the medically administered form when it is done at the patient's request. Legally, of course, there is a difference. An insurance company might refuse to pay off on a life policy in the case of self-administered euthanasia, calling it suicide. This fact is often presented as a legal-economic objection to euthanasia. It is not at all certain that because a coroner's jury finds a suicide was done "while of unsound mind" that the insurance benefits are thereby preserved. With the present moral philosophy of the law, wherein physical existence is the *summum bonum*, the higher intelligence which subordinates corrupted flesh to moral integrity will always appear unsound, so perhaps concern for insurance equities need not stay the patient's decision nor alarm his beneficiaries.

Bills to legalize euthanasia have been introduced without

success in the British Parliament in 1936 and in the state legislatures of Nebraska in 1937 and New York in 1947. The hurdle, of course, is partially ethical inertia and the cake of custom, partially legal prudence and timidity. The biggest issue is drawn around our ideas of murder. By general agreement murder is defined as "the killing of one human being by another *with malice aforethought*."[23] This definition is applied to condemn euthanasia when medically administered in just the same way that the concept of suicide is applied, as self-murder, when euthanasia is self-administered. The legal difficulty with any form of suicide, naturally, is that no sanction or penalty can be applied when the crime is successful. The law can operate only as a deterrent, since an attempt might be unsuccessful. "Although suicide is deemed a grave public wrong, yet from the impossibility of reaching the successful perpetrator, no forfeiture is imposed."[24] (Blackstone had approved burial in the highway, with a stake through the body and forfeiture of goods and chattels to the king.) Hence the remark of one Catholic moralist that euthanasia "is less honorable than the murder committed by a thug; the latter takes a chance on being caught and convicted."[25] But no such escape from penalty is open to the cooperating physician or friend in medical euthanasia. In the United States, at present, euthanasia is nowhere allowed by statute or by judicial decision. Some states, e.g., New York, hold that assisting a suicide is criminal. In Kansas, "every person deliberately assisting another in commission of self-murder shall be guilty of manslaughter in the first degree."[26] This reasoning is generally applied, equally, to those who help self-euthanasiasts, partake in suicide pacts, and make themselves parties to duels.

[23] 26 *American Jurisprudence*, 161.
[24] N.Y., sec. 2301, art. 202, bk. 39, McKinney's *Consolidated Laws of New York*.
[25] E. F. Burke, *op.cit.*, p. 55.
[26] Sec. 21-408, *General Statutes of Kansas*, 1929.

Moralists would contend that malice is not present as a motive in mercy-killings; that they are mercy-aforethought, not malice-aforethought. But a court, in Turner *v.* State, has ruled that hatred and malevolence are not necessary to express malice.[27] There need be only "an actual and deliberate intention to take the life of another." This makes malice in the law take on a technical meaning of premeditation, and when unqualified it makes euthanasia not only a felonious homicide but murder. For, unlike manslaughter, euthanasia is certainly a deliberated deed. The issue here is not a mere matter of legal precedents; it goes much deeper, to the philosophy of law and therefore to ethics and to our beliefs about human nature. As far as the law is concerned the problem may well center around the issue whether, ethically, the philosophy of law can rightly be satisfied with the doctrine that malice is implicit in the action of *felo de se.* This is a very questionable assumption indeed. There is some encouragement, therefore, in the recent discussions of English lawyers—precipitated by episodes of euthanasia—considering the advisability of making a rule that *express* malice must be established in order to determine guilt of murder.

Our courts already recognize and allow what they call justifiable homicide in some circumstances when we are attacked by other human beings. What the lawyers have not explained to the satisfaction of many interested moralists is why the same ethical elasticity may not be applied in cases of attack by disease and incurable suffering. Certainly the right to take life in self-defense is at stake in either situation. If it is replied that in self-defense against human attack we are seeking to preserve our life, whereas in euthanasia we are seeking to destroy our life, then we can and must call into question any such pure vitalism. We must deny that "life" is adequately understood as mere vital existence or breathing! For the man of moral integrity and spiritual

[27] Cited in *Linacre Quarterly,* 19.2, Apr. 1927.

purpose, the mere fact of being alive is not as important as the terms of the living. As every hero and every martyr knows, there are some conditions without which a man refuses to continue living. Surely among these conditions, along with loyalty to justice and brotherhood, we can include self-possession and personal integrity. Incurable pain destroys self-possession and disintegrates personality, as any wide acquaintance with sickbeds will teach us. Our medical servants know this only too well.

Furthermore, the law usually stipulates that murder is killing from a deliberate and premeditated design "unless it is excusable and justified."[28] Here is a legal qualification of the principle of malice which is highly apropos of euthanasia. It is a qualification made necessary in the law by such cases as the man who has had to plan his self-defense against someone with continuing but as yet unfulfilled designs on his life. Euthanasia is obviously planned and deliberate. It is precisely this that gives it its ethical quality! But it is also "excusable and justified" unless, of course, the law chooses to accept a purely vitalistic doctrine of man's being.

Perhaps the model legislation is to be found in a bill proposed in New York state by a committee of 1,776 physicians who want legislation to make euthanasia lawful, so that they and their patients may be protected from possible prosecution for a practice which, as everyone knows, goes on anyway. The bill is backed by the Euthanasia Society of America, and by thousands of doctors. It provides three things, essentially: (1) any sane person over twenty-one years old, suffering from an incurably painful and fatal disease, may petition a court of record for euthanasia, in a signed and attested document, with an affadavit from the attending physician that in his opinion the disease is incurable; (2) the court shall appoint a commission of three, of whom at least two shall be physicians, to investigate all aspects of the case and to

[28] Cf. C. F. Potter, *Readers Scope*, May 1947, p. 113.

report back to the courts whether the patient understands the purpose of his petition and comes under the provisions of the act; (3) upon a favorable report by the commission the court shall grant the petition, and *if it is still wanted by the patient* euthanasia may be administered by a physician or any other person chosen by the patient or by the commission.

There are elements in this proposal that deserve our thoughtful attention. The bill is permissive, not mandatory. Neither patient nor physician is compelled to act. The request for euthanasia must originate with the patient. The patient's freedom to change his mind at any time is fully guaranteed. Disinterested parties inquire into the whole matter. The permit is used only if and when the patient chooses. The proposal leaves aside the whole question of eugenic euthanasia for solution by some other legal instrument, since the merits of medical euthanasia are not inherently tied to the case for eugenic euthanasia.

Now that the United Nations has come into being, protagonists of euthanasia have carried their cause to that authority too. The terms of their appeals are much like those of the proposal to the New York State Assembly. They usually ask for an amendment to the Declaration of Human Rights which would include "the right of incurable sufferers to voluntary euthanasia," referring especially to Article Five of the Declaration, which states that "No one shall be subjected to torture." It is also pointed out that Articles Three and Eighteen declare that "everyone has the right to life, liberty, and *the security of person.* . . ." The right to life does not necessarily entail the obligation to live, especially when continued existence is so hideous and demoralizing that the *person* is blotted out and reduced to coma or ungovernable nerve-reactions. English advocates, who are in the thousands, have signed a petition to the United Nations. The list includes such persons as Sir J. J. Conybeare of Guy's

Hospital, London; Dr. Ernest Jones, president of the International Psychoanalytic Association; Julian Huxley, H. J. Fleure, G. E. Moore, Dean Inge, Canons Peter Green[29] and J. S. Bezzant; the Rev. Messrs. A. Herbert Gray, Donald Frazer, G. H. C. Macgregor and Hugh Martin; G. B. Shaw, Augustus John, Clifford Bax, Vera Brittain, Louis Golding, Kenneth Ingram, A. A. Milne, and R. Seebohm Rountree. Another recent convert to their ranks is Dean W. R. Matthews of St. Paul's, Inge's successor. Catholics are as clear as are non-Catholics that as far as law is concerned the issue of medical euthanasia is really one of judicial philosophy, not of mere precedent. In opposing legal euthanasia they would describe it as a question of theocentric versus anthropocentric morality. Those who use such question-begging neologisms (for such they really are, with or without any intention to avoid questions) would very probably characterize the freedom ethic running throughout this book as anthropocentric, although the correct problem is: given a theocentric context for the analysis of these matters, "What doth God require of thee?" How is that to be determined? In this particular case it is plain that many Christians do not find any theological logic (natural reason) or revelation to condemn euthanasia.

Pro and Con

It is at this point that we can turn to the definitely moral arguments for and against euthanasia. Our aim here is to be as orderly as possible in the discussion, and to forsake any *argumentum ad misericordiam*. We must try to avoid the penny-dreadful type of treatment Richard Cabot had in

[29] See Canon Green's short discussion in his *Problem of Right Conduct*, New York, 1931, pp. 283-284. This Anglican moralist says of euthanasia, "I have found it impossible to discover any really conclusive argument against suicide under due restrictions." See also in *Moral Problems*, ed. by the Bishop of Croydon, London, 1951, a permissive view taken by Lindsay Dewar, moral theologian of Bishop's College, and by the Bishop of Norwich.

mind when he spoke of euthanasia as "that ancient and reliable novelty . . . which the newspapers trick out afresh each year in August when politics are dull and there is a dearth of copy."[30] In a limited space, perhaps the best procedure will be to speak directly to the ten most common and most important objections. Therefore, suppose we deal with them as if they stood one by one in a bill of particulars.

1. It is objected that euthanasia, when voluntary, is really suicide. If this is true, and it would seem to be obviously true, then the proper question is: have we ever a right to commit suicide? Among Catholic moralists the most common ruling is that "it is never permitted to kill oneself intentionally, without explicit divine inspiration to do."[31] Humility requires us to assume that divine inspiration cannot reasonably be expected to occur either often or explicitly enough to meet the requirements of medical euthanasia. A plea for legal recognition of "man's inalienable right to die" is placed at the head of the physicians' petition to the New York State Assembly. Now, has man any such right, however limited and imperfect it may be? Surely he has, for otherwise the hero or martyr and all those who deliberately give their lives are morally at fault. It might be replied that there is a difference between the suicide, who is directly seeking to end his life, and the hero or martyr, who is seeking directly some other end entirely, death being only an undesired by-product. But to make this point is only to raise a question as to what purposes are sufficient to justify the loss of one's life. If altruistic values, such as defense of the innocent, are enough to justify the loss of one's life (and we will all agree that they are), then it may be argued that personal integrity is a value worth the loss of life, especially since, by definition, there is no hope of relief

---

[30] *Adventures on the Borderlands of Ethics, op.cit.,* p. 34.

[31] Davis, *op.cit.,* II, 142. This author explains that Jerome and Lessius excused suicide in defense of chastity, but that Aquinas opposed even this exception to the prohibition.

from the demoralizing pain and no further possibility of serving others. To call euthanasia egoistic or self-regarding makes no sense, since in the nature of the case the patient is not choosing his own good rather than the good of others.

Furthermore, it is important to recognize that there is no ground, in a rational or Christian outlook, for regarding life itself as the *summum bonum*. As a ministers' petition to buttress the New York bill puts it, "We believe in the sacredness of *personality*, but not in the worth of mere existence or 'length of days.' . . . We believe that such a sufferer has the right to die, and that society should grant this right, showing the same mercy to human beings as to the sub-human animal kingdom." (The point might be made validly in criticism of this statement that society can only recognize an "inalienable right," it cannot confer it. Persons are not mere creatures of the community, even though it is ultimately meaningless to claim integrity for them unless their lives are integrated into the community.) In the personalistic view of man and morals, asserted throughout these pages, personality is supreme over mere life. To prolong life uselessly, while the personal qualities of freedom, knowledge, self-possession and control, and responsibility are sacrificed is to attack the moral status of a person. It actually denies morality in order to submit to fatality. And in addition, to insist upon mere "life" invades religious interests as well as moral values. For to use analgesic agents to the point of depriving sufferers of consciousness is, by all apparent logic, inconsistent even with the practices of sacramentalist Christians. The point of death for a human person *in extremis* is surely by their own account a time when the use of reason and conscious self-commitment is most meritorious; it is the time when a responsible competence in receiving such rites as the viaticum and extreme unction would be most necessary and its consequences most invested with finality.

2. It is objected that euthanasia, when involuntary, is

murder. This is really an objection directed against the physician's role in medical euthanasia, assuming it is administered by him rather than by the patient on his own behalf. We might add to what has been said above about the word "murder" in law and legal definition by explaining that people with a moral rather than a legal interest—doctors, pastors, patients, and their friends—will never concede that malice means only premeditation, entirely divorced from the motive and the end sought. These factors are entirely different in euthanasia from the motive and the end in murder, even though the means—taking life—happens to be the same. If we can make no moral distinction between acts involving the same means, then the thrifty parent who saves in order to educate his children is no higher in the scale of merit than the miser who saves for the sake of hoarding. But, as far as medical care is concerned, there is an even more striking example of the contradictions which arise from refusing to allow for anything but the consequences of a human act. There is a dilemma in medication for terminal diseases which is just as real as the dilemma posed by the doctor's oath to relieve pain while he also promises to prolong life. As medical experts frequently point out, morphine, which is commonly used to ease pain, also shortens life, i.e., it induces death. Here we see that the two promises of the Hippocratic Oath actually conflict at the level of means as well as at the level of motive and intention.

3. What of the common religious opinion that God reserves for himself the right to decide at what moment a life shall cease? Koch-Preuss says euthanasia is the destruction of "the temple of God and a violation of the property rights of Jesus Christ."[32] As to this doctrine, it seems more than enough just to answer that if such a divine-monopoly theory is valid, then it follows with equal force that it is immoral

---

[32] *Op.cit.*, II, 76. He cites texts such as I Cor. 3:16-17.

to lengthen life. Is medical care, after all, only a form of human self-assertion or a demonic pretension, by which men, especially physicians, try to put themselves in God's place? Prolonging life, on this divine-monopoly view, when a life appears to be ending through natural or physical causes, is just as much an interference with natural determinism as mercifully ending a life before physiology does it in its own amoral way.

This argument that we must not tamper with life also assumes that physiological life is sacrosanct. But as we have pointed out repeatedly, this doctrine is a form of vitalism or naturalistic determinism. Dean Sperry of the Harvard Divinity School, who is usually a little more sensitive to the scent of anti-humane attitudes, wrote recently in the *New England Journal of Medicine* that Albert Schweitzer's doctrine of "reverence for life," which is often thought to entail an absolute prohibition against taking life, has strong claims upon men of conscience.[33] Perhaps so, but men of conscience will surely reject the doctrine if it is left unqualified and absolute. In actual fact, even Schweitzer has suggested that the principle is subject to qualification. He has, with apparent approval, explained that Gandhi "took it upon himself to go beyond the letter of the law against killing. . . . He ended the sufferings of a calf in its prolonged death-agony by giving it poison."[34] It seems unimaginable that either Schweitzer or Gandhi would deny to a human being what they would render, with however heavy a heart, to a calf. Gandhi did what he did in spite of the special sanctity of kine in Hindu discipline. In any case Dr. Schweitzer in his African hospital at Lambaréné is even now at work administering death-inducing-because-pain-relieving drugs. As William Temple once pointed out, "The

[33] Dec. 23, 1948. Incorporated in *The Ethical Basis of Medical Care*, op.cit., p. 160 sq.

[34] *Indian Thought and Its Development*, London, 1930, pp. 225-238.

notion that life is absolutely sacred is Hindu or Buddhist, not Christian." He neglected to remark that even those Oriental religionists forget their doctrine when it comes to *suttee* and *hara-kiri*. He said further that the argument that it cannot ever be right to kill a fellow human being will not stand up because "such a plea can only rest upon a belief that life, physiological life, is sacrosanct. This is not a Christian idea at all; for, if it were, the martyrs would be wrong. If the sanctity is *in* life, it must be wrong to give your life for a noble cause as well as to take another's. But the Christian must be ready to give life gladly for his faith, as for a noble cause. Of course, this implies that, *as compared with some things*, the loss of life is a small evil; and if so, then, *as compared with some other things*, the taking of life is a small injury."[35]

Parenthetically we should explain, if it is not evident in these quotations themselves, that Dr. Temple's purpose was to justify military service. Unfortunately for his aim, he failed to take account of the ethical factor of free choice as a right of the person who thus loses his life at the hands of the warrior. We cannot put upon the same ethical footing the ethical right to take our own lives, in which case our freedom is not invaded, and taking the lives of others in those cases in which the act is done against the victim's will and choice. The true parallel is between self-sacrifice and a merciful death provided at the person's request; there is none between self-sacrifice and violent or coercive killing. But the relevance of what Dr. Temple has to say and its importance for euthanasia is perfectly clear. The non-theological statement of the case agrees with Temple: "Are we not allowing ourselves to be deceived by our self-preservative tendency to rationalize a merely instinctive urge and to

[35] *Thoughts in War Time*, London, 1940, pp. 31-32. Italics in original.

attribute spiritual and ethical significance to phenomena appertaining to the realm of crude, biological utility?"[36]

4. It is also objected by religious moralists that euthanasia violates the Biblical command, "Thou shalt not kill." It is doubtful whether this kind of Biblicism is any more valid than the vitalism we reject. Indeed, it is a form of fundamentalism, common to both Catholics and reactionary Protestants. An outspoken religious opponent of euthanasia is a former chancellor to Cardinal Spellman as military vicar to the armed forces, Monsignor Robert McCormick. As presiding judge of the Archdiocesan Ecclesiastical Tribunal of New York, he warned the General Assembly of that state in 1947 not to "set aside the commandment 'Thou shalt not kill.' "[37] In the same vein, the general secretary of the American Council of Christian Churches, an organization of fundamentalist Protestants, denounced the fifty-four clergymen who supported the euthanasia bill, claiming that their action was "an evidence that the modernistic clergy have made further departure from the eternal moral law."[38]

Certainly those who justify war and capital punishment, as most Christians do, cannot condemn euthanasia on this ground. We might point out to the fundamentalists in the two major divisions of Western Christianity that the beatitude "Blessed are the merciful" has the force of a commandment too! The medical profession lives by it, has its whole *ethos* in it. But the simplest way to deal with this Christian text-proof objection might be to point out that the translation "Thou shalt not kill" is incorrect. It should be rendered, as in the responsive decalogue of the *Book of Common Prayer*, "Thou shalt do no murder," i.e., unlawful killing.

[36] H. Roberts, "Two Essays on Medicine," in *Living Age*, Oct. 1934, 347.159-162.

[37] Quoted H. N. Oliphant, *Redbook Magazine*, Sep. 1948.

[38] *Ibid.*

It is sufficient just to remember that the ancient Jews fully allowed warfare and capital punishment. Lawful killing was also for hunger-satisfaction and sacrifice. Hence, a variety of Hebrew terms such as *shachat, harag, tabach,* but *ratsach* in the Decalogue (both Exodus 20:13 and Deut. 5:17), clearly means *unlawful* killing, treacherously, for private vendetta or gain. Thus it is laid down in Leviticus 24:17 that "he who kills a man shall be put to death," showing that the lawful forms of killing may even be used to punish the unlawful! In the New Testament references to the prohibition against killing (e.g., Matt. 5:21, Luke 18:20, Rom. 13:9) are an endorsement of the commandments in the Jewish law. Each time, the verb *phoneuo* is used and the connotation is *unlawful* killing, as in the Decalogue. Other verbs connote simply the fact of killing, as *apokteino* (Luke 12:4, "Be not afraid of them that kill the body") and *thuo* which is used interchangeably for slaughter of animals for food and for sacrifice. We might also remind the Bible-bound moralists that there was no condemnation either of Abimelech, who chose to die, or of his faithful sword-bearer who carried out his wish for him.[39]

5. Another common objection in religious quarters is that suffering is a part of the divine plan for the good of man's soul, and must therefore be accepted. Does this mean that the physicians' Hippocratic Oath is opposed to Christian virtue and doctrine? If this simple and naive idea of suffering were a valid one, then we should not be able to give our moral approval to anesthetics or to provide any medical relief of human suffering. Such has been the objection of many religionists at every stage of medical conquest, as we pointed out in the first chapter in the case of anesthetics at childbirth. Here is still another anomaly in our mores of life and death, that we are, after much struggle, now fairly secure in the righteousness of easing suffering at birth but

[39] Judges 9:54.

we still feel it is wrong to ease suffering at death! Life may be begun without suffering, but it may not be ended without it, if it happens that nature combines death and suffering.

Those who have some acquaintance with the theological habit of mind can understand how even the question of euthanasia may be colored by the vision of the Cross as a symbol of redemptive suffering in Christian doctrine. As Emil Brunner has said of the crucifix, "it is not without its significance that the picture of a dying man is the sacred sign of Christendom."[40] But when it is applied to suffering in general it becomes, of course, a rather uncritical exemplarism which ignores the unique theological claims of the doctrine of the Atonement and the saving power of the Cross as a singular event. It is, at least, difficult to see how any theological basis for the suffering argument against medical euthanasia would be any different or any more compelling for keeping childbirth natural and "as God hath provided it."

It is much more realistic and humble to take as our regulative principle the rule that "Blessed are the merciful, for they shall see mercy," since this moral standard gives more recognition in actual fact to the motive of compassion, which, according to the theology of Atonement, lies behind the crucifixion of Jesus and gave it its power and its *ethos*. "All things whatsoever you would that men should do unto you, do you even so unto them." Mercy to the suffering is certainly the point of Psalm 102, vs. 12: "As a father hath compassion on his children, so hath the Lord compassion on them that fear him: for he knoweth our frame." Let the Biblicist take his position on the story of Job! Job explored the problem of human suffering and left it a mystery for the man of faith. Some have tried to find a recommendation of suicide in Job's wife's advice, but it is hardly more than

---

[40] *Man in Revolt*, New York, 1939, pp. 388-389.

a warning that he must not curse God.[41] In Job 7:15 there may be a thought of suicide, but nothing more than that. Our point here is that even Job never hinted that euthanasia was wrong; he only wondered, as we all do sometimes, why such a thing is ever needed or desired. The patience of Job is proverbial, but this is the Job of the prose part of the book. The poetry has another Job, a most rebellious and morally disturbed one. He could come to no other conclusion but that suffering is a mystery, as far as God's will and power are concerned. He did not give much attention to man's part in its control, nor to its particular aspect in incurable illness.

6. It is frequently pointed out, as an objection to euthanasia, that patients pronounced incurable might recover after all, for doctors can and do make mistakes. This seems, frankly, like a fundamentally obstructionist argument. It takes us back to the evasion based on fallibility with which we had to deal in the question of truth-telling. Doctors are indeed finite creatures. So they may also err in recommending and carrying out operations, or in other forms of treatment. As far as the accuracy of their advice is concerned, we have to trust them, although it is always our right to doubt their advice and to change doctors. If reluctance to trust them were a common attitude pervading medical relationships generally, it would spell the doom of medical care. Also, it is sometimes added that if we will just hang on something may turn up, perhaps a new discovery which will save us after all. Although this objection really evades the point at issue, it has a very great importance when seen in its own perspective. We always have ground for hope that many of the conditions which have called for euthanasia in the past will no longer do so. Not long ago crippling arthritis was thought almost hopeless, but cortisone and ACTH have offered new hope and success. Medical science is also continuously making discoveries which narrow the range of

[41] Job 2:9-10.

cases in which the conditions of justifiable euthanasia are apt to occur. Improved narcosis, new healing drugs and treatments, surgical relief of pain by new techniques of chordotomy and lobotomy—these things make news constantly.

And there are, of course, occasional incidents of totally unexpected, last-minute recovery from "hopeless" illnesses. An actual case would be that of the hospital chaplain who once stood by at a "certain" death and a horrible one from pemphigus. The doctors had even advised that the patient's family be called in for a last visit. Then, at the last moment, a new penicillin drug was flown in from another city, and the patient was saved. Such things happen, yes. But all we need to say to this objection to euthanasia is that by no stretch of the imagination, in a typical situation, can we foresee a discovery that will restore health to a life already running out. A patient dying of metastatic cancer may be considered already dead, though still breathing. In advanced cases, even if a cure were to be found, toxemia has in all likelihood damaged the tissues and organs fatally.

7. It is said, with some truth, that patients racked by pain might make impulsive and ill-considered requests for euthanasia, if it were morally and legally approved. To this there are two rejoinders: first, that a careful law, such as that of the Euthanasia Society, would provide that there must be medical advice that death is certain, which rules out any hasty euthanasia in non-fatal illnesses; and, second, that the law would provide an interval between application and administration. The law should not permit euthanasia to be done on the spur of the moment, and the patient should be free to withdraw his request at any time. The requirement that the disease must be of a fatal character is needed to guard against unconscious wishes for destruction which are to be seen sometimes, although rarely, in patients. The confirmation of the patient's and the attending physician's

decisions by disinterested parties is a sufficient bulwark against impulsive action. This might also be the place to emphasize that a doctor is always free to refuse to administer medical euthanasia, as a patient ought to be free to request it. In a wide search of the literature, incidentally, only one really *medical* objection to the practice was found, although there are frequent moral objections. Dr. A. A. Brill, of the International Psychoanalytical Association, has declared that *although doctors are actually doing it they should stop*, because for reasons of depth psychology the practice will demoralize both patients and doctors, fill them with fear that inhibits healing relationships and lowers vitality.[42] As we have already seen, Dr. Brill's colleague in the Association, Dr. Ernest Jones, does not regard this as a real objection to euthanasia, if we may draw that conclusion from his support of it before the United Nations.

Connected with this is this further objection: what if the patient can no longer speak or even gesture intelligibly? Can we be sure we always understand the patient's real desire, his choice for or against death, especially in cases where his condition is nearly unconscious or comatose? We all know that communication is not solely verbal. The provision that the request must come from the patient in a documentary form is introduced in proposals like that of the Euthanasia Society out of great caution, presumably in the fear that a gesture or other sign might be misinterpreted. A restriction like this will also exclude the possibility of a doctor's carrying out euthanasia when the patient had expressed a desire for it but the formalities could not be fulfilled before his physical powers to apply had failed. This would be tragic, but perhaps it is the necessary price exacted for legalization. There is also, of course, the reverse possibility that a patient might make the proper application, then change his mind after his powers of communication

42 *Journ. of Nervous and Mental Diseases*, July 1936, p. 84.

had failed. But these seem unreal problems, purely logical in character, if it is held, as we indeed do hold, that a patient who has completely lost the power to communicate has passed into a submoral state, outside the forum of conscience and beyond moral being. Being no longer responsive, he is no longer responsible.

Conscience and consciousness are inseparable and presuppose each other. Their interdependence has always been recognized, since the Stoics first explored the cognitive aspect of conscience as distinct from the judicial, and recognized that to act with *conscientia*, with knowledge, requires consciousness. The Stoics predicated awareness or consciousness of Natural Law insight; the Christians have predicated Natural Law insight plus communion with God and the voice of the Holy Spirit. Some have held that the moral factor in consciousness is innate; others, acquired. Some have thought it to be reason; others, intuition; still others, emotion. In any case, these faculties are parts of consciousness, without which personality is gone and there is no longer a "person" to fulfill even the minimum requirements of moral status, i.e., freedom and knowledge.

8. Sometimes we hear it said that the moral and legal approval of euthanasia would weaken our moral fiber, tend to encourage us to minimize the importance of life. Hence such well-known witticisms as G. K. Chesterton's, that the proponents of euthanasia now seek only the death of those who are a nuisance to themselves, but soon it will be broadened to include those who are a nuisance to others.[48] It is very hard to find any real hope of taking hold of an objection like this, with its broad value-terms such as "moral fiber" and "the importance of life." It could just as easily be reasoned that to ask for euthanasia, to leave voluntarily for the unknown, would call for courage and resolution and faith, and would encourage us to live with faith and without

---

[48] Symposium, "Pro and Con," in *The Digest*, Oct. 23, 1937, 124.22-23.

fear of the unknown. There is great wisdom and moral assurance in the decision of Charlotte Perkins Gilman, one of
America's greatest women, who chose self-euthanasia rather
than endure a degenerative death by cancer. These were her
last words, typed by her own hand: "A last duty. Human
life consists in mutual service. No grief, no pain, misfortune or 'broken heart' is excuse for cutting off one's life
while any power of service remains. But when all usefulness is over, when one is assured of an imminent and unavoidable death, it is the simplest of human rights to choose
a quick and easy death in place of a slow and horrible one.
Public opinion is changing on this subject. The time is
approaching when we shall consider it abhorrent to our
civilization to allow a human being to lie in prolonged
agony which we should mercifully end in any other creature.
Believing this choice to be of social service in promoting
wider views on this question, I have preferred chloroform
to cancer."[44]

Our attention should be given particularly to one sentence
here: "No grief, no pain, no misfortune or 'broken heart' is
excuse for cutting off one's life while any power of service
remains." It is a cause for joy that many avenues of service
are open, or could be opened, to properly diagnosed terminal
patients. Because of its psychological effects, genuine service,
or being needed, will postpone the unendurable stages of
pain or collapse. Enlightened hospital procedure is making
great advances in this respect. One of the most significant
services open to terminal patients is willingness to submit
to drugs and cures and narcotics of an experimental kind,
aimed at eliminating *the very pain and demoralization which
is a major justification for euthanasia.* This consideration is
certainly a welcome one to the advocates of euthanasia, and
is always kept in mind by them. For them the best possible

[44] Quoted by A. L. Woolbarst, *Medical Record*, May 17, 1939.

news would be that medicine has at last deprived euthanasia of its *raison d'être*.

Sometimes it is suggested by advocates of euthanasia that those who insist that the suffering go on are unconscious sadists, moved by the wish to make others suffer, or in a voyeurist version actually eager to see them suffer. This is an extremely problematical ground upon which to enter in the discussion, and it tends to "psychologize" all ethical reason out of the picture. It is true, theoretically, that the idea of noble suffering may be, deep down, a reaction-formation to rationalize sadistic or masochistic sentiments. But on the other hand, opponents of euthanasia could charge that the advocates are the victims of a death instinct or destruction-wishes; or even a sado-masochist syndrome, sadist in the friends of the patient, masochist in the patient. To this, in their turn, the advocates could reply that if they were sadistic in their drives they would *want* the suffering to go on. There are hardly any limits to the kind of wool-gathering that could develop along these lines, with little or no possibility of contributing to a solution ethically.

9. It is objected that the ethics of a physician forbids him to take life. We have already recognized that fact *as a fact*, but the issue is raised precisely because there are cases when the doctor's duty to prolong and protect life is in conflict with his equal duty to relieve suffering. As a matter of fact, this dilemma is actually inescapable and inherent in the medical care of many terminal illnesses anyway, at the technical as well as the moral level. If the physician's obligation is both to relieve pain and prolong life, how then can he use analgesics, which bring relief but have the necessary effect of hastening death? Great strides in non-toxemic medications are being made, but it remains true that, for example, prolonged morphine has a lethal effect, especially when finally there is a failure of natural functions such as breathing, salivation, and heat regulation, and when it no

longer works intravenously because circulation is ceasing and it has to be injected directly into the heart. Everyone concerned in the care of the sick knows quite well that the medication itself is euthanasia. We hear constantly of overdoses somehow or other taken in terminal cases. There are many cases indeed in which actions are carried out by patients or attendants in the spirit of Socrates, drinking the cup of hemlock, who cried to Crito, "We owe a cock to Aesculapius. . . . Pay the debt and do not forget it."[45]

The dilemma of the physician who takes a contradictory oath could hardly be more evident than in the words of an article in *The New England Journal of Medicine* entitled "The Theology [sic] of Medicine." The author, a physician, declared, "I feel as Dr. Woodward did when he said, 'I have no sympathy with the man who would shorten the death agony of a dog but prolong that of a human being.' "[46] Dr. Woodward had himself advised a class of medical students, "I hold it to be your duty to smooth as much as possible the pathway to the grave even if life is somewhat shortened. Nor is it necessary to talk it over with friends and relatives, nor need you expect them to formally countenance either neglect or expedition. Let that be your affair, settled with your own conscience."[47] It is a dilemma. The only real problem in conscience is not whether the mystique of vitalism or an ethic of mercifulness should reign, but whether the decision should rest upon the lonely conscience of the doctor without honest approval or responsibility shared fully with patient and family. Dr. Woodward is correct ethically to show mercy, but he is not justified in being so god-like about it. He should be man-like about it, and so should the students to whom he was giving his advice. As long as doctors continue, as at present, making unilateral decisions, they are in

[45] *Phaedo*, conclusion.
[46] R. E. Osgood, M.D., 210.4, 182-192, Jan. 25, 1934.
[47] *Ibid.*, 202.18, 843-853.

the position of needing something stronger than a Rule of Double Effect of their own, whereby they can convince themselves that it is right to do a good thing if they do not intend the evil consequences. Under these circumstances, can they sort out their emotions and motives, and make sure that they do not *want* the luckless patient to reach an end to his sufferings? Under these circumstances, what of the Hippocratic Oath?

Our defense of the right to die, with the doctor's aid, is not made in any kind of illness except the fatal and demoralizing ones. Besides, as we have seen in other questions already discussed, there are common exceptions to the rule against medical homicide. If one can be made at the beginning of life (abortion) why not also at the end of life (euthanasia)? The one situation is no more absolute than the other. There is no more stigma in the one than in the other. On personalistic grounds we could say that there is less question morally in euthanasia, for in euthanasia a merciful death is chosen in cooperation with a person whose integrity is threatened by disintegration, whereas an embryo in therapeutic abortion has no personal value or development at stake and cannot exercise the moral qualities of freedom and knowledge.

10. Finally, it is objected that doctors do not want euthanasia made legal.[48] It is not at all uncommon to hear doctors admit that they generally engage in the practice, in one way or another. Lest any reader be skeptical, he should examine the Cumulative Book Index and the index of periodicals for medical opinion on the subject, and he will find several places in which the admission is candidly made.[49] From

[48] Cf. G. E. Byers, *Ohio Med. Journ.*, 1936, 32.342; J. S. Manson, *Brit. Med. Journ.*, 1936, 1.86; W. W. Gregg, *North Amer. Rev.*, 1934, 237.239; J. J. Walsh, *The Forum*, Dec. 1935, 333-334. The Council of the World Medical Association, at Copenhagen, Apr. 24-28, 1950, *recommended* that "the practice of euthanasia be condemned." Cf. *Journal of the Amer. Med. Assoc.*, June 10, 1950, 143-6, p. 561.

[49] E.g., cf. Frank Hinman, M.D., *Journ. of Nervous and Mental Diseases*, 99, 1944.

time to time there are reports, undocumentable but from usually reliable sources, of medical meetings such as one recently in the Middle West at which a speaker asked for a show of hands from those who have never administered euthanasia. Not a hand was raised.[50] In 1935 great excitement was caused by a doctor's public confession in a London newspaper that he had been practicing euthanasia, and in *Time Magazine* an article reported, "Pungent, voluble Dr. Morris Fishbein, editor of the American Medical Association's *Journal*, observed that the average doctor frequently faces the problem, that when it is a matter between him and his patient he may decide it in his own way without interference."[51] Many are the uses which we may be sure are made of drugs such as bichloride of mercury, potassium cyanide, and some of the barbiturates. In 1947, when an English doctor publicly announced he too engaged in medical euthanasia, a spokesman for the British Medical Association, in a very oblique but patent *non dixit*, said, "I think a good many doctors feel as Dr. Barton does, that euthanasia ought to be legalized. The association has no objection to doctors saying what they think about law."[52]

There are three other objections closely allied to these we have examined. They may deserve just a word or two. First, it is said that medical euthanasia would weaken medical research, that it would take away the incentive to find cures for painful maladies. This is nonsense because doctors are already practicing euthanasia and yet their fight against fatal diseases is mounting, not flagging. As cancer and malignant tumors, for example, increase (nearly 200,000 Americans will die of them this year) the research in that field increases too. The motive behind medical research is the elimination or control of disease, not merely the avoidance of

[50] Cf. H. N. Oliphant, *op.cit.*
[51] Nov. 18, 1935, 26.21, pp. 53-54.
[52] *New York Herald Tribune*, May 23, 1947.

suffering.[53] Second, it is objected that the heirs or enemies of an invalid might use euthanasia to hasten his death. To this we reply that the legal requirement of a written application by the sufferer, and of both legal and medical investigations, would be a safeguard. He would have far more protection than is provided for many patients now committed for treatment of mental disorder. He would, indeed, have a great deal more protection than he now receives under the present system of clandestine euthanasia being widely practiced. Third, it is claimed that once we legalize mercy deaths the application of the principle will be widened disastrously to cover non-fatal illnesses. But why is it, then, that although legal killing by capital punishment has been in vogue a long time, yet it has been narrowed rather than extended in scope? In fact it has been narrowed a great deal from the days when people were hanged for stealing a few shillings. This alarmist objection is the old red herring against which we have had to aim the rule of *abusus non tollit usum* time and again. It is drawn across many ethical trails.

A Time to Plant, a Time to Pluck

To draw our thinking together, we ought to repeat that there are three schools of thought favoring euthanasia. First, there are those who favor voluntary euthanasia, a personalistic ethical position. Second, there are those who favor involuntary euthanasia for monstrosities at birth and mental defectives, a partly personalistic and partly eugenic position.[54] Third, there are those who favor involuntary euthanasia for

[53] See the thrilling story of vigorous medical progress in an account by the Secretary of the American Medical Association, Stephen M. Spencer, *Wonders of Modern Medicine*, New York, 1953. Between 1900 and 1952 the average life span of Americans has risen from 49 to 69 years, and Louis I. Dublin of the Metropolitan Life Insurance Company estimates it will be 73 within this generation, thus exceeding the threescore and ten allotted in the Bible.

[54] It has always been a quite common practice of midwives and, in modern times, doctors, simply to fail to respirate monstrous babies at birth.

all who are a burden upon the community, a purely eugenic position. It should be perfectly obvious that we do not have to endorse the third school of thought just because we favor either the first or the second, or both. Our discussion has covered only the first one—voluntary medical euthanasia— as a means of ending a human life enmeshed in incurable and fatal physical suffering. The principles of right based upon selfhood and moral being favor it.

Defense of voluntary medical euthanasia, it should be made plain, does not depend upon the superficial system of values in which physical evil (pain) is regarded as worse than moral evil (sin) or intellectual evil (error). On the contrary, unless we are careful to see that pain is the least of evils, then our values would tie us back into that old attitude of taking the material or physical aspects of reality so seriously that we put nature or things as they are *out there* in a determinant place, subordinating the ethical and spiritual values of freedom and knowledge and upholding, in effect, a kind of naturalism. C. S. Lewis has described it by saying that, "Of all evils, pain only is sterilized or disinfected evil."[55] Pain cannot create moral evil, such as a disintegration or demoralization of personality would be, unless it is submitted to in brute fashion as opponents of euthanasia insist we should do.

We repeat, the issue is not one of life or death. The issue is which kind of death, an agonized or peaceful one. Shall we meet death in personal integrity or in personal disintegration? Should there be a moral or a demoralized end to mortal life? Surely, as we have seen in earlier chapters, we are not as persons of moral stature to be ruled by ruthless and unreasoning physiology, but rather by reason and self-control. Those who face the issues of euthanasia with a religious faith will not, if they think twice, submit to the materialistic and animistic doctrine that God's will is re-

[55] *The Problem of Pain*, London, 1943, p. 104.

vealed by what nature does, and that life, qua life, is absolutely sacred and untouchable. All of us can agree with Reinhold Niebuhr that "the ending of our life would not threaten us if we had not falsely made ourselves the center of life's meaning."[56] One of the pathetic immaturities we all recognize around us is stated bluntly by Sigmund Freud in his *Reflections on War and Death*: "In the subconscious every one of us is convinced of his immortality." Our frantic hold upon life can only cease to be a snare and delusion when we objectify it in some religious doctrine of salvation, or, alternatively, agree with Sidney Hook that "the romantic pessimism which mourns man's finitude is a vain lament that we are not gods."[57] At least, the principles of personal morality warn us not to make physical phenomena, unmitigated by human freedom, the center of life's meaning. There is an impressive wisdom in the words of Dr. Logan Clendenning: "Death itself is not unpleasant. I have seen a good many people die. To a few death comes as a friend, as a relief from pain, from intolerable loneliness or loss, or from disappointment. To even fewer it comes as a horror. To most it hardly comes at all, so gradual is its approach, so long have the senses been benumbed, so little do they realize what is taking place. As I think it over, death seems to me one of the few evidences in nature of the operation of a creative intelligence exhibiting qualities which I recognize as mind stuff. To have blundered onto the form of energy called life showed a sort of malignant power. After having blundered on life, to have conceived of death was a real stroke of genius."[58]

As Ecclesiastes the Preacher kept saying in first one way and then another, "The living know that they shall die" and there is "a time to be born and a time to die, a time to

---

[56] *Human Destiny*, New York, 1943, II, 293.
[57] Quoted by Corliss Lamont, *The Illusion of Immortality*, New York, 1950, p. 191.
[58] *The Human Body*, New York, 1941, 3rd ed., pp. 442-443.

plant and a time to pluck up that which is planted."[59] And in the New Covenant we read that "all flesh is as grass" and "the grass withereth, and the flower thereof falleth away." Nevertheless, "who is he that will harm you, if ye be followers of that which is good?"[60]

Medicine contributes too much to the moral stature of men to persist indefinitely in denying the ultimate claims of its own supreme virtue and ethical inspiration, mercy. With Maeterlinck, we may be sure that "there will come a day when Science will protest its errors and will shorten our sufferings."[61]

[59] Eccl. 9:5 and 3:2.
[60] I Pet. 1:24 and 3:13.
[61] Quoted by Jacoby, op.cit., p. 206.

CHAPTER SEVEN

THE ETHICS OF PERSONALITY: MORALITY, NATURE, AND HUMAN NATURE

WHY not call to order *what is over against us*, and send it packing into the realm of objects? . . . And in all the seriousness of truth, hear this: without *It* man cannot live. But he who lives with *It* alone is not a man."[1] Physical nature—the body and its members, our organs and their functions—all of these *things* are a part of "what is over against us," and if we live by the rules and conditions set in physiology or any other *it* we are not men, we are not *thou*. When we discussed the problem of giving life to new creatures, and the authority of natural processes as over against the human values of responsibility and self-preservation (when nature and they are at cross-purposes), we remarked that spiritual reality and moral integrity belong to man alone, in whatever degree we may possess them as made *imago Dei*. Freedom, knowledge, choice, responsibility—all these things of personal or moral stature are in us, not *out there*. Physical nature is what is over against us, out there. It represents the world of *its*. Only men and God are *thou*; they only are persons. And ethical insight and moral status are the qualities of personality alone. As Seward Hiltner once said, "We surely do well to state as bluntly and often as possible that what *is* . . . has thereby no normative significance."[2] What is simply given in nature has no moral value; it is without *character* since it neither exerts nor requires any moral choice or decision.

[1] Martin Buber, *I and Thou*, op.cit., p. 34.
[2] In *Sex and Religion*, ed. by Doniger, op.cit., p. 13.

But we should hasten to say that this is not the whole truth. It would be wrong to give the impression that nature, in our own human physique or in any other part of the natural order, is merely indifferent material to be used or discarded without respect to its constitution, its limits, order, and trend. We must repeat that man is himself a creature of the natural order. He cannot be autonomous. William Temple expresses the relationship helpfully: "Nature is man's partner rather than his servant." However, the context for Temple's statement is the habit in some social systems of exhausting the natural resources which are vital to human society, for the sake of selfish private profit or in a prodigal disregard of supply. "The treatment of the earth by man the exploiter is not only imprudent but sacrilegious."[3] Our context is another one. Man's relation to his own physical frame is one of partnership too. And while his body, with its powers, is not a mere servant, to be manipulated and ordered about as having no claims or worth of its own, neither is it an overlord of man. In a partnership there is give and take. If men and women have to bow down before nature's ways to the extent of giving up life or health in involuntary parenthood, or of submitting to intolerable and futile suffering in terminal illnesses, or of submitting to childlessness in cases of sterility, or of denying the sexual function provided by nature itself when ethical objections to procreation exist, then the body has become the master. It is no longer a partner. And in the last analysis the analogy has to break down, anyway, for ethical reasons, since a partnership must be entered into by two or more "competent persons." But the body is *it*. It is not a person, nor is it morally competent, necessary though it may be as the basis of human personality. A much better analogy lies in the artist and his materials: man the artist, the body the materials. A good artist loves and respects his materials, but

[3] *The Hope of a New World*, New York, 1943, p. 67.

he is the artist always. Even so, "no man ever hates his own flesh, but nourishes and cherishes it."[4]

Our ethic rightly rests upon a principle of freedom within responsibility. This entails two negative *oughts*: (1) we ought not to submit willy-nilly to what is, to physical and physiological facts simply as they are, since to do so would be to be unfree; and (2) we ought not to ignore or disregard or flout what is, simply because it is unchosen, since to do so would be to be guilty of an unrealistic denial of human finitude and creaturehood and therefore irresponsible—toward both our natural necessities and our social obligations.

There is a measure of important truth in the evolutionary conception of ourselves, of course. The basic matter of our bodies rises to a higher form in our life or vitality (what St. Paul called *psyche* or soul), and life rises to a higher form in consciousness or mind, and mind rises to a higher form in the spirit (what St. Paul called *pneuma*). Animals too have mind, consciousness. But theirs is an *instinctual* consciousness. It is not rational or critical. Animals cannot possess themselves of real knowledge, nor can they exercise real choice. Their values are given in their physical frame and the nature around them. They can choose only between the means to ends or purposes that are already fixed and determined for them by instinct. In short, they are not persons. But men, the spiritual or moral creatures, can and do choose between ends as well as between means. Men select their goods and suit the means to them accordingly. Unlike the lower animals, men, because they are moral beings or persons, know the difference between good and evil. This is both their glory and their tragedy, that they are "condemned to be free." Before the dawn of conscience they were like the brutes who still remain, ethically, in the Garden of Eden. They were then unmoral brutes. But for

4 Eph. 5:29.

better or for worse they are persons now, with all the moral responsibility of personal status. This is the radical difference between man and that nature with which he lives and moves and shares his being. Self-consciousness marks the frontier between *thou* and *it*. Therefore men cannot be guided by what unconscious nature does. They alone can discern the values which qualify their relation to physical nature. Their eyes are opened and they are "as gods knowing good and evil."

All along we have presented a case for the moral approach to problems of health and life and death, as over against the natural standard of what is medically good and evil. We have often expressed this case as the personal versus the physical, or physiological, standards of morality. Deliberately we have relied upon a cumulative support for our central thesis, choosing to bring out what it means in a clinical style by examining concrete problems rather than by presenting a contrived and systematic construction of ethical doctrine. It is better, after all, to let doctrine weave itself in and out of real life and practical questions in medical care. In the end, all ethical issues are concrete. We have to say our yes or no to existing choices; we cannot judge in the abstract.

Certain things have emerged from this process. The criteria of moral status, of genuine personality, have reasserted themselves persistently and time after time. Fundamentally they are the two basic postulates always present in ethics, (a) freedom of choice and (b) knowledge of the things between which to choose. Our grasp of them is never complete, but without them any talk of morality is meaningless. This freedom is opposed, in medical care, to the physiological *status quo* and the dictates of natural law. This knowledge is opposed to the cultural *status quo*, and the dictates of customary morality or the cake of custom. To accept this principle means inevitably that we have to part firmly with any attempt to assign to nature personal qualities and character traits such as intentions and rights and moral integrity. We have seen what it means *not* to do so in matters of conception, pregnancy, disease, inheritable defects, and fatal suffering. It means also that biology cannot provide the content of theology. There is no possible ground for supposing that a scrutiny of nature's ordinary and average phenomena can reveal either the will of God or a norm for men. It repudiates, for example, a naive vitalism which would make life more valuable than *living by spiritual standards*, and which prefers to maintain life at the cost of demoralization and depersonalization. It means, also, rejecting a natural law which demands submission to the amoral cause-and-effect of biological procreation without regard for the higher values of voluntary and creative parenthood. Our principle of personal integrity, on the other hand, asserts that there is a place for the doctrine of human agency in the scheme of creation, which is a process as well as an event. In any ethical outlook of religious faith, men are people and not puppets. It is a false humility or a subtle determinism which asks us to "leave things in God's hands." The worst forms of determinism and fatalism are spiritualistic, not materialistic. They are more often grounded in theistic religion than in humanism. Perhaps this is why the devil is a spiritual figure, representing spiritual wickedness in high places!

We might use one final illustration to show the degree to which naturalistic determinism of medical morals has managed to fetter the consciences of conscientious men. The issue was a debate in 1948 between Geoffrey Fisher, the Archbishop of Canterbury, and a majority of the House of Lords. In a divorce case (Baxter *v.* Baxter) the husband had asked for a nullification of his marriage on the ground of non-consummation, charging that his wife had refused intercourse except with the use of contraceptives.[5] The lords were agreed that procreation is not the sole validating end of marriage. The Archbishop, on his side, however, claimed that "consummation, which means completion, has not been reached, if, by the use of artificial means, procreation has been wilfully and deliberately prevented." He was altogether positive in his opinion that "it is a Christian duty of a man and wife, unless prevented by *physical* means, to have children." We have no reason to doubt that His Grace was entirely sincere in believing that he held parenthood to be the primary purpose of marriage. No doubt he *thought* that he regarded children as the real validation of marriage. But does he? In August of the same year the Archbishop declared that A.I.D. is an act of adultery, and that this means therefore that it provides grounds in canon law as well as in civil law for divorce of the marriage bond! It becomes clear that in actual fact the Archbishop does not hold that children and parenthood are uppermost in value. The decisive factor to validate a marriage, in his reasoning, is the morally indifferent pattern of natural processes. It is natural law that is uppermost in his hierarchy of values. For although he holds that a man and wife must seek to procreate, he first predicates of their effort that it must be done according to the terms and conditions and limitations set by brute physiology and biology. Whether blind nature happens to hasten or to hinder, to provide or deny parenthood, he would have us submissively bow to its happenstance. Thus far and thus fundamentally do men of good will often make good an unmoral determinant and will a mockery!

We have seen how many religious moralists are concerned above all with the alleged supernatural rights of souls, whereas our own priority goes to personality, to the person. What is the difference? What is a person? Why should we

[5] *The Witness*, Feb. 19, 1948; *New York Times*, Mar. 17, 1948; also *New York Times*, July 17, 1945 and Dec. 18, 1947.

assert so boldly that medical care at a high ethical level is person-centered; that it should correct for its tendency to be preoccupied with diagnosis since the discoveries of Virchow and Pasteur? Why should it not be *soul*-centered? We can put our position very simply and quite directly. Ethics is not concerned with souls for the simple reason that "soul" is neither a spiritual nor a moral value! Our presuppositions can be expressed, if one chooses, in the language of Biblical theology. This question of a soul in reality has nothing to do with the issues between a religious and a humanist view of human nature. To use the terms of Professor Moss, an Anglican theologian, "man is made up of three parts, closely connected together. The material part of man belongs to the animal kingdom in the material world. Man is a living being, and therefore has, besides his body, *a life or soul, which other animals have too.* But he is also spirit, as well as soul and body: which the other animals are not."[6] The soul of man in primitive culture, like the *nephesh* or *psyche* in Biblical literature, is nothing more than the animation of the psychophysical organism, its vital principle. It is what makes him, and all the other animals, tick and be alive.

In the creation myth, the soul is the body activated by God's breath, as in Genesis 2:7. And St. Paul in his essay on eternal life, in I Corinthians 15, distinguishes between the body born as *psychikon soma* (or "soul-ish" body, which is the natural body of mortality "sown in corruption") and the nurtured person of the *pneumatikon soma* (or spiritual body, which is "raised in incorruption," capable of saying yes or no to the invitation to eternal life). Throughout most of the Bible the soul is life or self. Thus in Matthew 16:25-26 and its parallel in Mark 8:35-36, the words "soul" and "life" are interchangeable in the Authorized Version. But in the

---

[6] C. B. Moss, *The Christian Faith: An Introduction to Dogmatic Theology,* New York, 1943, p. 135. Cf. a supporting Biblical explanation in Millar Burrow's *Outline of Biblical Theology,* Philadelphia, 1946, pp. 134-141. Italics added.

Revised Standard Version, the scholars have made "life" the word of translation in every case. "For what will it profit a man if he gains the whole world, and forfeits his *life?* Or what shall a man give in return for his *life?*" The point is that in any case when he dies his soul will be lost, but his self may be saved. The soul is not a pre-existent *something* that is put into the person from outside, whether by a direct gift of God in a creationist manner or by transmission through our parents in a traducian manner. All of this soul-doctrine and soul-oriented morality is a pre-scientific, pre-psychological anthropology. It is, furthermore, a Greek idea not to be found in Hebrew or Biblical thought. It leads to pagan beliefs in immortality as an inherent quality of human being, and to fearsome prospects of heaven or hell in the life after death. The New Testament faith in eternal life is in resurrection, according to which the person or self can be spiritually raised from mortality by God's doing and not through any quality of the person himself. This is a totally different faith in which the alternatives after death are life through resurrection of the spirit, or extinction. The very word "soul" is in the same dubious, murky condition that we have found in the term "natural law." It is too obscure, not to say obscurantist, to deserve any further use in either common-sense or Christian ethics.

We are concerned primarily with man's spiritual quality and his selfhood. It is the integrity of the personality that has first claim in the forum of conscience. To be a person, to have moral being, is to have the capacity for intelligent causal action. It means to be free of physiology! It means to have selfness or self-awareness. This is something that is not found in the body or in any of its organs. In Biblical terms it means that man is made in the image of God, and that therefore he is self-conscious, saying "I am," and that he is self-determined, saying "I will." However imperfectly and finitely, he is nevertheless a person, as God is a person who said of himself, "I am that I am." This is what it means to be a person and not an object to be manipulated either by doctors of medicine or by the impassive operations of physical nature. In a strict use of language, St. Paul is utterly wrong to say that "there is no respect of persons with God."[7] It may be true, of course, as St. Paul really meant to say, that God has no special or discriminatory concern for personages set apart in our human rivalries for social status and prestige. But it is precisely persons—and not souls or bodies or glands or human biology—that count with God and come first in ethics.

None of this is to be taken by humano-romantics as putting the person of man in God's place. Men are still men— finite, self-deceptive, failing even when they succeed at their task of being loyal to their moral stature. As we have already seen, the ethical effect of scientific conquests may well be to put them to immoral as well as to moral uses. An increase of man's control over the means and ends of human living does indeed increase his moral stature, but it also puts into his hands a know-how with which he may do greater rather than less evil. But men, as men, are as yet only neophytes in the spiritual world and the forum of conscience. Their possession of a central nervous system and brain capacity equal to the functions of conscience is so recent, compared to the long history of men before Eve ate the apple, that *moral* men have existed figuratively for only fifteen minutes or less out of the human day. Change and growth are the rules of his moral being. There are those who feel that men are worse than ever before, what with wars and atom bombs and genocide, but they fail to understand that it is the more powerful *means* that produce the greater evils. The terrible differential is scientific, in our instrumentalities; not moral, in the disposition of our wills, our attitudes. As to good will in men, it is probably no less

[7] Rom. 2:11.

than it was a hundred years ago, while it is perceptibly greater than it was a thousand years ago and infinitely greater than ten thousand years ago. As far as moral standards and ethical values are concerned, who can doubt that the mores of health and community and respect for persons have increased in the broad secular trend in the direction of altruism and mercy? We can substitute our focus on medical morality for the social system in this quotation from Hastings Rashdall: "Who can doubt that many features of our existing social system are equally (with slavery) incompatible with the principles of Christ's teaching, and that the accepted Christian morality of a hundred years hence will definitely condemn many things which the average Christian conscience now allows?"[8]

At this point there will be those who say indulgently, "You cannot change human nature." This has always been the slogan of anti-rational philosophy and conservative politics. Science knows better. Anthropology knows that human nature has assumed the most diverse and improbable forms, all the way from the Zuñis' distaste for personal success and distinction to the nerve-wracking and nerve-wrecking competition for social status in present-day American culture; all the way, again, from the polygamy and incest of the ancient Old Testament people to the strict monogamy of latter-day Christian marriage. Just as we have found that it is necessary to lay aside the notions of natural law and soul because they stand in the way of ethical medical care, so we may find that we have to lay aside the notion of man, about whom so many reactionary, dogmatic, and absolute claims are being made. Emil Brunner gets far enough to ask the question, "Is it true that 'man' as such exists at all?"[9] Brunner manages somehow to find man by asserting that all men are personal or have personality. So far, so true. But

[8] *Philosophy and Religion*, New York, 1910, p. 166.
[9] *Man in Revolt*, New York, 1939, p. 38.

when we examine this personality, Brunner discovers that it is only what Aristotle quite sensibly meant in his doctrine of the rational faculty of self-possession. On any view, all the way from an Aristotle to a Ralph Linton, there is no reason to regard this personality of men as fixed, static, predetermined. Actually, there is no ground left for this ancient idea of man-stuff; no ground is left except a literary or liturgical one for asking with the Psalmist, "What is *man* that thou art mindful of him?" On the contrary, the medical and social sciences have shown that the personalities of men are culture-tied and conditioned by a host of social and physical but variable factors.

What, then, can the modern philosopher mean when he speaks of "the essential nature of man," in ethics or in any other field of inquiry? Can he mean that men enter into their historically conditioned existence with a certain hard core of being, a human *stasis,* around which all relative traits are gathered? Certainly not! It seems plain enough that he can only mean this: that men in a vast majority of instances *acquire* certain common traits called personality which are not characteristic of other creatures. One such high-incidence trait, and the foundation of our moral status, is rational (conceptual) understanding, with its capacity for critical action.

Theologically speaking, this is to say that personality is not created by divine *fiat,* but by a divinely ordained process of development in human organisms, just as human self-consciousness is itself a relatively late emergent in the whole evolutionary process. Men thus *become* persons; they actually have to assemble their qualities of personal stature developmentally. They may be described as "made in the image of God," but that cannot mean that the image or likeness is manufactured by God prior to their psychophysical birth and growth. God is indeed the maker of men, but only indirectly, because he has ordered all things and all things come of him.

To oppose this modern view of man would be to embrace of necessity some notion of the soul and to end up in antiquarian ideas of the soul's infusion at the moment of conception or some time later in the fetus. It would put men in the same category with the unconditioned being of God, or at the least make them half-gods and half-men. But the sober truth is that men are indeed actually finite, not-God. And even in terms of natural theology it should be plain that God creates them as emergents rather than by *fiat* or special creation. To imagine that men's special importance presupposes a special creation is to commit the genetic fallacy of judging the worth or value of a thing by its origin, rather than by its achievement.

All these considerations follow from a study of health, life, and death in medicine and morals. But perhaps the most important insight we gain is that ethical integrity cannot compromise with any naturalistic doctrine, whether it be in the form of vitalism or determinism. We need not repeat that the counter-Reformation version of the classical Natural Law, which in its new form so consistently subordinates human values to the law of nature, is a perversion of a moral norm into a physical or material norm. In its practical applications to medical care it comes too close to naturalistic ethics to be tolerated, and this is because it tends to assert that what nature "does," on the average, is *ipso facto* good. As G. E. Moore expressed it, "If everything natural is equally good, then certainly ethics, as it is ordinarily understood, disappears: for nothing is more certain, from an ethical point of view, than that some things are bad and others good."[10] In the same way that a dubious syllogism lies behind the claim that contraceptive birth control is against nature, so there is a similar fault in any other employment of fatality thinking. The major premise of all naturalistic ethics, whether Father Slater's, Nietzsche's, or Herbert Spencer's,

[10] *Principia Ethica*, New York, 1939, p. 42.

in effect becomes the proposition that whatever is natural is good. It suggests that whatever situation at any time exists is good; that whatever is, is good. This is meaningless in ethics, if not in every other forum. Going by nature is anti-moral when going by nature's ways is made the norm, for to follow such a norm is to forsake the imperative mood for the indicative mood, and to convert ethics from an enterprise in value-judgments into a descriptive discipline aimed at making human actions coincide with natural, i.e., given, conditions. When nature rules, conscience is made of none effect and reduced to the amoral level of natural cause and effect, that is, *non compos mentis*.

None of this is directed against the principle of ethical realism. But it is a defensible opinion that the classical concept of Natural Law has been too discredited by perversions of the sort we have met in the ethics of medical care to permit any further use of the term. Something else—perhaps "moral order"—is better and may more pointedly set itself apart from the fatalism that thinks of the Natural Law as the "laws of nature." Our own position can be stated succinctly by using a previous statement, taken somewhat out of context but legitimate here because of its endorsement of ethical realism as against any form of naturalism, relativism, or positivism: "Is there a moral order, objectively existent, to which both individuals and the law of the community are subordinate? Is morality a part of reality? Does the law formulate and enforce justice and right, or does it create them? Is a thing right because the law says so, or does the law say so because it is right? . . . In our humblest moods, as rational creatures we all have to have answers to these bedrock questions of human existence. It is this writer's conviction that there *is* a moral order; that we seek it but we do not make it. Medieval and ancient moralists called it the Natural Law; religionists call it the Will of God; our American founding fathers, in the Declaration of Independence, called it 'certain unalienable rights.' Whatever name we give it, it is there. Morality is an aspect of what is, as well as an ideal of what ought to be."[11] This ethical realism is an article of faith, even though at the same time we have to be ethical relativists as far as knowledge is concerned, knowing that our ethical values are always subject to correction by fresh experience and capable of greater depth and scope as science, technology, and social progress increase our insights and add to our power of control over self and over the external world.

There is urgent reason for trying to develop our understanding of medicine and morals, and for deepening our ethical insights. Were medical workers and non-Catholics to expend the care and concern we have seen in the studies of the Roman theologians, how much might be gained for man's moral stature and for the claims of mercy and well-being! With the one stellar exception of Catholic moralists there is a strange blindspot about the ethics of health and medicine in almost all ethical literature. Volume after volume in general ethics and in religious treatises on morality will cover almost every conceivable phase of personal and social ethics except medicine and health. It is high time that we brought our ethical and spiritual experience, and its new dimensions of understanding, to bear upon the care of the sick in the same deliberate and creative way that psychology has been explored and applied for the sake of those who are ill and in need of counsel and treatment. The appearance in recent years of pastoral psychology in the work of ministers should be fortified by an equivalent pastoral ethics in order that justice may be as well served as adjustment, in the same way that medical psychology in general should be buttressed by a more rational medical morality. The morality of medicine is fully as incumbent upon us all as the psychology of medicine. But to accomplish the task creatively

11 Joseph Fletcher, in *Social Meaning of Legal Concepts: Criminal Guilt*, New York, 1950, pp. 175-176.

and constructively, it will have to be required of religious moralists that they clear their path of all otiose dogmas which contribute to the stultifying influences of customary morality. This should not be as difficult as cleaning the Augean Stables. And yet as an example of how easily moralists can turn their most glorious convictions into stumbling blocks, when they do not take care, we can quote again from Rashdall: "The most deadly result of the doctrine of justification by faith, whether in its extreme Reformation expressions or any other of its cruder forms, is that it has fostered the belief that honest thinking is sinful, and that there is merit in blind credulity. . . . Its deadly fruit still poisons the religious life of the average parish or congregation. It deters the clergy from study, from thought, and from openly teaching what they themselves really believe. It prevents the cooperation of Christians with one another and with others, who without fully sharing the Christians' belief, to a large extent share the same practical aims."[12]

The possibilities of "breadth, and length, and depth, and height" in the morals of medicine are almost limitless. To such an enterprise much can be brought not only by the ethically sensitive of all stripes of opinion and diverse backgrounds, but in many ultimate respects there are factors of special value and importance to be brought by theological moralists. As *curatores animarum* they have a long history of concern and involvement with the practical aspects and human episodes of health, life, and death.[13] Let them order their going in the way with the wise and realistic words of Thomas à Kempis. "Whilst thou art in health, thou canst do much good; but I know not what thou wilt be able to do when ailing. There are few who mend their ways in sickness, just as those who go much on pilgrimage seldom become holy."[14]

[12] *The Idea of Christian Atonement*, London, 1919, pp. 428-429.
[13] For a recent historical account, cf. J. T. McNeill, *A History of the Cure of Souls*, New York, 1951.
[14] *Imitatio Christi*, I, I, c.23.

BIBLIOGRAPHY
AND
INDEX

SELECTED BIBLIOGRAPHY

Works having a bearing on the morals of medicine, historically as well as critically, are much too numerous to be listed. The following selection of books, chiefly critical, will indicate the thoroughgoing nature of Roman Catholic studies, the relative scarcity of scientific and general studies, and the virtual non-existence of Protestant literature.

GENERAL ETHICAL WORKS

Paul Blanshard, *American Freedom and Catholic Power*, Boston, 1949.

J. H. Breasted, *The Dawn of Conscience*, New York, 1934.

Martin Buber, *Between Man and Man*, New York, 1948.

R. C. Cabot, *Adventures on the Borderland of Ethics*, New York, 1926.

Gerald Heard, *Morals since 1900*, New York, 1950.

G. W. Jacoby, *Physician, Pastor and Patient*, New York, 1936.

Halliday Sutherland, *Laws of Life*, New York, 1936.

Eduard Westermarck, *Christianity and Morals*, New York, 1939.

SCIENTIFIC WORKS

R. C. Cook, *Human Fertility: the Modern Dilemma*, New York, 1951.

Josué de Castro, *The Geography of Hunger*, Boston, 1952.

A. F. Guttmacher, *Life in the Making*, New York, 1933.

H. H. Haggard, *Devils, Drugs and Doctors*, New York, 1929.

J. H. Landman, *Human Sterilization: the History*, New York, 1932.

Lynn Thorndike, *A History of Magic and Eyperimental Science*, New York, 1923-41.

A. D. White, *The History of the Warfare of Science with Theology*, New York, 1897.

PROTESTANT WORKS

Simon Doniger, *Sex and Religion Today*, New York, 1953.

J. P. Hinton and J. E. Calcutt, *Sterilization: A Christian Approach*, London, 1935.

Daniel Jenkins, *The Doctor's Profession*, London, 1949.

John T. McNeill, *A History of the Cure of Souls*, New York, 1951.

F. F. Rigby, *Problems of Personal Relationships*, London, 1952.

Willard Sperry, *The Ethical Basis of Medical Care*, New York, 1950.

ROMAN CATHOLIC WORKS

A. Bonnar, *The Catholic Doctor*, London, 1937.

T. L. Bouscaren, *Ethics of Ectopic Operations*, Chicago, 1933.

E. F. Burke, *Acute Cases of Moral Medicine*, New York, 1922.

F. J. Connell, *Morals in Politics and Professions*, Westminster, Md., 1946.

Henry Davis, *Artificial Human Fecundation*, New York, 1951.

Henry Davis, *Moral and Pastoral Theology* (Vol. ii), New York, 1943.

B. J. Ficarra, *Newer Ethical Problems in Medicine and Surgery*, Westminster, Md., 1951.

P. A. Finney, *Moral Problems in Medical Practice*, St. Louis, 1922.

Dom Peter Flood, *New Problems in Medical Ethics*, Westminster, Md., 1953.

W. K. Glover, *Artificial Insemination Among Human Beings: Medical, Legal and Moral Aspects*, Washington, 1948.

F. L. Good and O. F. Kelley, *Marriage, Morals and Medical Care*, New York, 1951.

O. Griese, *The Morality of Periodic Continence*, Washington, 1942.

R. J. Huser, *The Crime of Abortion in Canon Law*, Washington, 1942.

Gerald Kelley, *Medico-Moral Problems*, St. Louis, i, 1949; ii, 1950; iii, 1951.

A. Klarman, *The Crux of Pastoral Medicine*, New York, 1905.

Stanislas Larochelle, *Handbook of Medical Ethics for Nurses, Physicians and Priests*, Westminster, Md., 1943.

C. J. McFadden, *Medical Ethics*, Philadelphia, 1949.

Austin O'Malley, *The Ethics of Medical Homicide and Mutilation*, New York, 1919.

BIBLIOGRAPHY

Walter Reaney, *The Creation of the Soul*, New York, 1932.

A. E. Sanford, rev. W. M. Drum, *Pastoral Medicine: A Handbook for the Catholic Clergy*, New York, 1905.

J. V. Sullivan, *Catholic Teaching on the Morality of Euthanasia*, Washington, 1949.

INDEX

233

INDEX

INDEX

INDEX

INDEX

INDEX

INDEX

Walsh, J. J., 23, 205

war, 27, 60, 69, 100-3, 109, 129, 131, 158, 195, 219

Washburn, F. H., 6

water subcut, 51

Westermarck, Eduard, 130, 147, 179

White, A. D., 23-4

Whitehead, A. N., xiii

Whitman, Walt, 170

White House Conference on Child Health and Protection, 141

wills, 50

Wilson, Woodrow, 71

witch doctor, 3

Woodward, S. B., 204

Woolbarst, A. L., 202

Worcester, Alfred, 9, 53

Wordsworth, William, 94

World War II, iv, 128, 139

x-ray tubes, 26

xenophobia, 29

Yale University, 16

Zilpah, 119

Zimri, 178

Zoar, 130

Zuñis, 220